Case Studies in Abnormal Child and Adolescent Psychology

To my students at Denison

Sara Miller McCune founded SAGE Publishing in 1965 to support the dissemination of usable knowledge and educate a global community. SAGE publishes more than 1000 journals and over 800 new books each year, spanning a wide range of subject areas. Our growing selection of library products includes archives, data, case studies and video. SAGE remains majority owned by our founder and after her lifetime will become owned by a charitable trust that secures the company's continued independence.

Los Angeles | London | New Delhi | Singapore | Washington DC | Melbourne

Case Studies in Abnormal Child and Adolescent Psychology

Robert Weis

Denison University

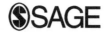

Los Angeles | London | New Delhi
Singapore | Washington DC | Melbourne

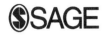

FOR INFORMATION:

SAGE Publications, Inc.
2455 Teller Road
Thousand Oaks, California 91320
E-mail: order@sagepub.com

SAGE Publications Ltd.
1 Oliver's Yard
55 City Road
London, EC1Y 1SP
United Kingdom

SAGE Publications India Pvt. Ltd.
B 1/I 1 Mohan Cooperative Industrial Area
Mathura Road, New Delhi 110 044
India

SAGE Publications Asia-Pacific Pte. Ltd.
18 Cross Street #10-10/11/12
China Square Central
Singapore 048423

Acquisitions Editor: Abbie Rickard
Editorial Assistant: Elizabeth Cruz
Production Editor: Bennie Clark Allen
Copy Editor: Christina West
Typesetter: Hurix Digital
Proofreader: Sue Schon
Cover Designer: Scott Van Atta
Marketing Manager: Katherine Hepburn

Printed in Canada

Library of Congress Cataloging-in-Publication Data

Names: Weis, Robert, 1973- author.

Title: Case studies in abnormal child and adolescent psychology/Robert Weis, Denison University.

Description: Los Angeles : SAGE, [2021] | Includes bibliographical references.

Identifiers: LCCN 2020025075 | ISBN 9781071808146 (paperback ; alk. paper) | ISBN 9781071808160 (epub) | ISBN 9781071808177 (epub) | ISBN 9781071808184 (epub)

Subjects: LCSH: Child psychopathology–Case studies. | Adolescent psychopathology–Case studies.

Classification: LCC RJ499 .W3923 2021 | DDC 618.92/89–dc23

LC record available at https://lccn.loc.gov/2020025075

This book is printed on acid-free paper.

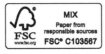

20 21 22 23 24 10 9 8 7 6 5 4 3 2 1

CONTENTS

HOW TO USE THIS BOOK

Case Studies in Abnormal Child and Adolescent Psychology is a collection of clinical vignettes designed to accompany the fourth edition of the textbook *Introduction to Abnormal Child and Adolescent Psychology*. The cases are organized according to the structure of the textbook, which reflects the meta-structure of the *Diagnostic and Statistical Manual of Mental Disorders*, Fifth Edition (DSM-5). The first section presents cases that illustrate principles of developmental psychopathology, psychological assessment, and evidence-based treatment. The remaining sections present neuro-developmental disorders, disruptive behavior disorders and substance use problems, emotion and thought disorders, and health-related conditions, respectively.

Each vignette is presented briefly (one or two pages) and reflects an actual child, adolescent, or family with names and other identifying information changed to protect their confidentiality. Cases are followed by a series of discussion questions that correspond to material presented in the text. The questions invite students to critically evaluate or apply principles of developmental psychopathology, describe key diagnostic features of each disorder, identify potential causes for children's problems from multiple levels of analysis, and/or formulate treatment plans based on empirical evidence.

This text includes instructor teaching materials, including suggested answers to the case materials. These are designed to save you time and to help you keep students engaged. To learn more, visit **sagepub.com** or contact your SAGE representative at **sagepub.com/findmyrep**.

Instructors can use these case studies in several ways:

As In-Class Activities

Because the vignettes are short, you can present a case to your entire class at the beginning of the class session. Then, after presenting material relevant to that vignette, you can ask your students to apply what they have learned at the end of the session.

For Class Presentations or Group Projects

Alternatively, you can assign cases to groups of students ahead of time. Each group might be responsible for presenting their case to the rest of the class and/or addressing the discussion questions you want to emphasize. Oral presentations can be relatively brief (i.e., 5–10 minutes each) and might be given periodically during the semester or as an end-of-semester project.

Another strategy is to set aside a class session for "grand rounds." You can assign each group a vignette in a common theme (e.g., communication disorders, anxiety disorders, mood disorders) and ask groups to present their case to the class. This strategy is particularly effective for helping students differentiate among similar disorders or notice common causes or treatments for different disorders.

As Writing Assignments or Exam Questions

Of course, each case study could be presented either as a writing assignment or exam question. As writing assignments, cases give students opportunities to review, evaluate, and apply information from the text. As exam questions, they allow you to assess students' mastery of material at a deeper level of processing than most short-answer or multiple-choice questions.

Perhaps most importantly, these vignettes help students to focus on *children and families*, rather than on disorders. I hope that these case studies give you greater freedom to engage and challenge your students in new and creative ways. If you have other ideas that have worked well for you, and are willing to share, I'd love to hear them!

Robert Weis

Denison University

Granville, Ohio

weisr@denison.edu

CONCEPTS, METHODS, AND THEORIES

THE SCIENCE AND PRACTICE OF ABNORMAL CHILD PSYCHOLOGY

CASE STUDY

WHAT IS ABNORMAL?

Mental health professionals have long struggled with the best way to differentiate mental disorders from mental health. The DSM-5 conceptualization of mental disorders borrows heavily from Jerome Wakefield's (1992) notion of "harmful dysfunction." According to Wakefield, disorders reflect an 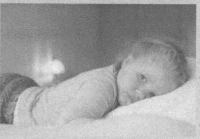 underlying biological or psychological dysfunction that causes harm to the individual. The DSM-5 definition of a mental disorder is reproduced below:

> A mental disorder is a syndrome characterized by clinically significant disturbance in an individual's cognition, emotion regulation, or behavior that reflects a dysfunction in the psychological, biological, or developmental processes underlying mental functioning. Mental disorders are usually associated with significant distress or disability in social, occupational, or other important activities. An expectable or culturally approved response to a common stressor or loss, such as the death of a loved one,

(Continued)

(Continued)

is not a mental disorder. Socially deviant behavior (e.g., political, religious, sexual) and conflicts that are primarily between the individual and society are not mental disorders unless the deviance or conflict results from a dysfunction in the individual, as described above. (American Psychiatric Association, 2013, p. 20)

Read each of the following brief case studies. Using the DSM-5 definition above, determine if the child in each case study has a mental disorder. If there's not enough information in the case study, identify any other information you would need to determine if the child meets the DSM-5 definition.

1. Margaret wets the bed at night. She does not wake up until the next morning. Her parents spend a great deal of time and energy washing her pajamas and bedding.

2. Shawn is afraid to ride elevators. Every time he is in an elevator, he experiences intense feelings of panic. He tries to avoid elevators whenever he can.

3. Charlotte is a teenage girl whose father died of a heart attack. Charlotte isn't eating or sleeping well. She can't concentrate on her homework or activities at school. Sometimes, at night, she talks with her father about her day before she falls asleep. She also thinks a lot about death.

References

American Psychiatric Association. (2013). *Diagnostic and statistical manual of mental disorders* (5th ed.). Washington, DC: Author.

Wakefield, J. (1992). Disorder as harmful dysfunction. *Psychological Review, 99,* 232–247.

This case study accompanies the textbook: Weis, R. (2021). *Introduction to abnormal child and adolescent psychology* (4th ed.). Thousand Oaks, CA: Sage. Answers appear in the online instructor resources. Visit **https://sagepub.com**.

CASE STUDY

ETHICAL DILEMMAS WITH CHILDREN AND FAMILIES

Researchers surveyed psychologists about ethical dilemmas that they encountered in their practice. Some of the most common problems involved (1) questions about maintaining confidentiality, (2) potential conflicts of interest, (3) when and how to provide informed consent, and (4) practicing within one's boundaries of competence (Pope & Vasquez, 2016).

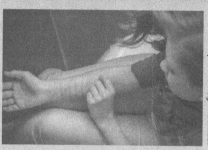

©iStockphoto.com/grummanaa5

Ethical issues are especially difficult in psychotherapy with children and families. The American Psychological Association's (2017) ethics code can help psychologists resolve ethical dilemmas. Read each of the following ethics scenarios. Identify the ethical principle that is most relevant to the scenario. Then use this ethical principle to determine how you might act in that situation.

Ethics Scenario 1: You are a therapist in private practice who has been providing counseling to Aimee, a 15-year-old girl with anxiety and depression. Over the last few weeks, Aimee's symptoms have worsened and she has admitted to cutting herself. Her mother wants to know what is wrong. What should you do to act in an ethical manner?

Ethics Scenario 2: You are an undergraduate psychology major who is participating in an internship at a residential treatment facility for adolescents with conduct problems. One of the social workers at the facility asks you to lead a group therapy session with several residents each week. The focus of the therapy session will be to help the adolescents develop emotion regulation and social skills. What should you do?

Ethics Scenario 3: You are a behavior therapist working at a special needs preschool. You've been assigned to work with Meredith, a 6-year-old girl who has low intellectual functioning and autism spectrum disorder. Meredith becomes angry and tantrums when she must brush her teeth or her hair in the morning. Your task is to reduce the frequency and severity of these tantrums. What must you do to proceed in an ethical manner?

Ethics Scenario 4: You are a psychologist working at a local high school. One of your friends, a teacher at the high school, asks you to help her daughter, a 14-year-old middle school student who has been acting very depressed and withdrawn in recent weeks. After meeting with the girl for a few sessions, you learn that she is sexually active and may be pregnant. What must you do to act in an ethical manner?

(Continued)

(Continued)

References

American Psychological Association. (2017). *Ethical principles of psychologists and code of conduct*. Washington, DC: Author.

Pope, K. S., & Vasquez, M. J. (2016). *Ethics in psychotherapy and counseling: A practical guide*. New York, NY: Wiley.

This case study accompanies the textbook: Weis, R. (2021). *Introduction to abnormal child and adolescent psychology* (4th ed.). Thousand Oaks, CA: Sage. Answers appear in the online instructor resources. Visit **https://sagepub.com**.

THE CAUSES OF CHILDHOOD DISORDERS

Developmental psychopathology is a multidisciplinary approach to understanding normal and abnormal development over the lifespan. It conceptualizes development in terms of risk and protective factors that place individuals on developmental pathways toward adaptation or maladaptation (Cicchetti & Rogosch, 2002).

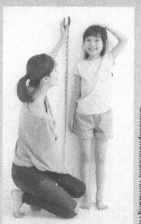

©iStockphoto.com/Tomwang112

Developmental psychopathologists are interested in continuity versus change across development. Almost a century ago, Sigmund Freud wrote about the difficulty in predicting children's development over time:

> So long as we trace development from its final outcome backwards, the chain of events appears continuous. . . . But if we proceed the reverse way, if we start from the premises and try to follow these up to the final result, we notice at once that there might have been another result and we might have been just as well able to understand and explain the latter. Hence the chain of causation can always be recognized with certainty if we follow the line of analysis backwards, whereas to predict it is impossible. (Sroufe & Rutter, 1984)

(Continued)

(Continued)

Read the following scenarios and answer each question. What principle of developmental psychopathology does each scenario illustrate?

1. Carlos is a 14-year-old boy with a long-standing history of attention-deficit/hyperactivity disorder (ADHD). He began to show problems with hyperactivity and impulsivity as a preschooler. In early elementary school, he also began exhibiting poor attention and concentration. Now in the eighth grade, Carlos continues to show all of these symptoms. He manages these symptoms with medication and behavioral interventions administered by his parents and teachers.

   What principle of developmental psychopathology does Carlos illustrate?

2. Haley is a 17-year-old high school student with a history of separation anxiety disorder. When Haley was a toddler, she followed her parents around the house and cried when they left her with a babysitter. Haley refused to attend preschool and was resistant to begin kindergarten when she turned 6 years old. In early elementary school, Haley's separation anxiety decreased, but she continued to worry about "bad things" happening to her parents when she was separated from them.

   Now in high school, Haley reports no significant problems with separation anxiety. However, in the past 6 months, she has experienced several panic attacks—intense episodes of fear characterized by rapid heart rate, shallow breathing, and intense distress. Her pediatrician confirmed that these attacks are not caused by a medical problem. Her mother has sought help from a psychologist who specializes in adolescent anxiety disorders.

   What principle of developmental psychopathology does Haley illustrate?

3. The juvenile court in one county hears cases for approximately 75 youths and families each month. Although the children who appear before the court come from different backgrounds and have different histories, they almost always show problems with antisocial behavior or substance use.

   What principle of developmental psychopathology does this scenario illustrate?

4. Adeba is a social worker who is employed by Child Protective Services. Adeba is assigned a new case, an 11-year-old girl who experienced repeated sexual abuse by her stepfather. Adeba wants to determine the girl's prognosis, but she can't predict the girl's future with much certainty.

   What principle of developmental psychopathology does she illustrate?

References

Cicchetti, D., & Rogosch, F. A. (2002). A developmental psychopathology perspective on adolescence. *Journal of Consulting and Clinical Psychology, 70*, 6–20.

Sroufe, L. A., & Rutter, M. (1984). The domain of developmental psychopathology. *Child Development, 55*, 17–29.

This case study accompanies the textbook: Weis, R. (2021). *Introduction to abnormal child and adolescent psychology* (4th ed.). Thousand Oaks, CA: Sage. Answers appear in the online instructor resources. Visit **https://sagepub.com**.

CASE STUDY

BIO-PSYCHO-SOCIAL CAUSES OF CHILDREN'S PROBLEMS

Just like the characters in *The Blind Men and the Elephant*, we obtain the most complete picture of children's development (and developmental problems) when we look at it from multiple perspectives. Developmental psychopathologists study childhood disorders across multiple levels of analysis: biological, psychological,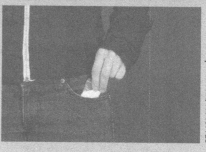

and social–cultural. Then, they combine information from across these levels to explain how disorders emerge over time.

Now it's your turn to apply the various levels of analysis presented in the text to a clinical case. Read the case study and briefly explain how Valerie's disorder can be explained in terms of each level, and how the levels might interact with each other, over time, to shape development.

Description

Valerie Connell was a 16-year-old girl who was referred to an inpatient residential treatment program for adolescents with substance use disorders. Val was ordered to participate in treatment by the juvenile court after she was arrested for opioid possession and distribution.

Val grew up in a western suburb of Chicago. Her father was a musician with a history of alcohol and marijuana use problems. He left Val and her mother when Val was 5 years old. Although he continued to live in the Chicago area, he had only occasional contact with Val. Val had mixed feelings about her father. On one hand, she was attracted to his glamorous lifestyle: performing, traveling, and socializing. On the other hand, she resented his decision to abandon his family when she was so young and harbored anger toward him because of the many times he disappointed her over the years. "If your own dad doesn't care about you, no one will," said Val. "I saw myself as pretty worthless—like no one will ever really love me."

Val's mother also had a history of alcohol use. She became pregnant with Val when she was 17, a single parent by the time she was 22, and a recovering alcoholic by the time she was 26. Mrs. Connell attends Alcoholics Anonymous meetings to maintain her sobriety and supports herself and Val by working two jobs. Long hours limit her ability to be involved in Val's school or extracurricular activities. Although she says, "Val means the world to me—the one thing I live for," she admits that stress at work and concerns about her ability to pay the bills "sometimes cause me to lose my temper with her."

Val exhibited problems with hyperactivity and oppositional behavior as a preschooler. "She was a handful," recalled her mother. "She'd always be on the go,

(Continued)

(Continued)

she never wanted to be quiet and listen to me. If I would tell her to do some-thing, she'd ignore me, yell, or scream." Val's disruptive behavior persisted into elementary school. Her pediatrician prescribed stimulant medication to manage her hyperactive-impulsive behavior, but it had little effect on her defiance and tan-trums. By the time Val was in the third grade, she was behind her classmates in reading and math and had gained a reputation as a troublemaker.

Val's substance use began with her transition to middle school. She was referred to a special education program for children with behavior problems and learning disabilities. She quickly made friends with several girls who introduced her to smoking (age 12) and marijuana (age 13). Although she tried alcohol at approximately the same age, she did not like its taste and limited its use to parties and social gatherings. By the time Val was 14 years old, she was using marijuana several times per week and drinking five to six sweet alcoholic drinks at parties on the weekends. She found it easy to hide her substance use from her mother.

Val transitioned to an alternative high school during her freshman year. "All of the kids there used drugs," Val recalled. Her 17-year-old boyfriend introduced her to prescription pain medication. Val's favorite combination was OxyContin in the morning followed by Roxicodone periodically throughout the school day. She quickly became known as the "Oxy and Roxy" girl. "I'd sleep during class, slur my speech, didn't care about anything," she recalled. "The teachers didn't say any-thing to me because I didn't cause trouble, so I kept on going." Val obtained $10 pills from her boyfriend and sold them to classmates for $25, pocketing the profits to support her own drug use.

"I first used heroin with my boyfriend—a different boyfriend—during my sopho-more year," Val reported. "I was afraid of needles so I snorted it. The feeling was excellent, like all the pain in my life was taken away. I could relax, stay still, and not worry about school or family. Snorting worked much faster than taking pills and the effects of heroin were much better." Within 6 months, Val was using heroin approximately 3 times per day to sustain its positive effects and avoid withdrawal symptoms such as anxiety, nausea, and agitation. Her use became expensive and she engaged in prostitution several times to support her habit.

"It might seem crazy, but I'm kind of glad that I got caught," Val reported. "I've been to the funerals of two friends who died from heroin. My life was on the wrong track." In residential treatment, Val was prescribed a medication called Subox-one, a combination of buprenorphine (an opiate substitute that reduces cravings) and naloxone (a medication that blocks the positive effects of heroin). The physi-cian and psychologist at the residential treatment facility hope that it will help her reduce her opioid use (see Fiellin et al., 2014).

"I'm not sure what I'm going to do when I get out of here," reported Val. "My mom wants me to come back home, but I can't go back. Everyone I know uses. I need a clean break."

Discussion Questions

1. How might you explain Val's substance use disorder in terms of behavioral genetics and epigenetics?

2. How might you explain Val's problems with (a) hyperactivity-impulsivity and (b) substance use in terms of the brain and neurotransmitters?

3. How might you use learning theory to explain Val's substance use disorder?

4. How might problems with cognition or emotion regulation contribute to Val's substance use problems?

5. How might Val's parents and peers contribute to her substance use problems?

6. How might social–cultural factors contribute to Val's substance use problem?

Reference

Fiellin, D. A., Schottenfeld, R. S., Cutter, C. J., Moore, B. A., Barry, D. T., & O'Connor, P. G. (2014). Primary care–based buprenorphine taper vs maintenance therapy for prescription opioid dependence: A randomized clinical trial. *JAMA Internal Medicine, 174*(12), 1947–1954.

This case study accompanies the textbook: Weis, R. (2021). *Introduction to abnormal child and adolescent psychology* (4th ed). Thousand Oaks, CA: Sage. Answers appear in the online instructor resources. Visit **https://sagepub.com**. This case is based on interviews conducted by Paul Grondahl for the *Albany Times Union*.

CASE STUDY

BUTTERFLY DI: A CASE OF GENE–ENVIRONMENT CORRELATION

Scarr and McCartney's (1983) notion of gene–environment correlation can be used to explain the way genotype and environment affect each other to shape development. Chapter 2 in the text presents the case study of Kirby, a boy with emerging disruptive behavior problems. However, gene–environment correlation can also be applied to children 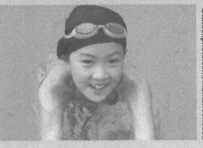 whose development seems to be coming along "swimmingly." Read the case study below and identify how the theory of gene–environment correlation can be applied to Diana's development.

Description

Diana was born to swim. Her mother was an Olympic athlete whose relay medley team won the bronze medal in Atlanta. Today, Diana's mother is the head swim coach at a Division II college in Diana's hometown. Although Diana's father was not a swimmer, he was a Division I baseball player who currently works as a personal trainer. Diana also has two older sisters who earned college scholarships for swimming and diving, respectively.

Diana was a healthy baby who enjoyed all of the benefits of a health-conscious family. Her father, who studied nutrition in college, was extremely conscientious about his family's eating habits. Diana and her sisters ate a largely vegetarian diet and received excellent medical care. Her mother decorated Diana's room in an aquatic theme: blue walls, fish-patterned bedsheets, an octopus pillow, and a dolphin nightlight.

Diana began taking swim lessons at the age of 18 months. She was more agile in the pool than on land. Her mother would swim with her and her sisters several times per week. Diana also attended her older sisters' swim lessons and, later in her childhood, she would also attend their swim meets.

Diana began to swim competitively at the age of 5 for a summer aquatic league. By the time she was 7, she was swimming year-round for a 10-and-under recreational team at the YMCA and winning many of her events. One of the coaches recognized her raw talent and invited her to join his travel team that practiced at the local college. Diana joined the team several months later, practiced 5 days per week, and received individual lessons from the head coach.

Diana swam on the varsity team during her freshman year of high school. She excelled in all events, especially the butterfly. Diana bonded with other girls on the team and had success in the pool and in the classroom.

Now 17-year-old Diana is beginning her final year as a high school swimmer. A shoulder injury sustained in a car accident earlier in the year slowed down her stroke and probably eliminated her chances of a Division I scholarship. However, Diana has visited several Division III schools with excellent swimming programs that would provide her with a good education and an opportunity to swim competitively for 4 more years. "Swimming's not the only thing important in my life, but it's a major part of it," Diana said. "I can't imagine giving it up just yet."

Discussion Questions

1. How does Diana illustrate passive gene–environment correlation?

2. How does Diana illustrate evocative gene–environment correlation?

3. How does Diana illustrate active gene–environment correlation?

Reference

Scarr, S., & McCartney, K. (1983). How people make their own environments: A theory of genotype environment effects. *Child Development, 54*, 424–435.

RESEARCH METHODS WITH CHILDREN AND FAMILIES

Many years ago, researchers conducted one of the most ambitious studies designed to investigate whether we could prevent juvenile delinquency in at-risk youths. The research project was funded by a retired professor of social ethics and medicine named Richard Cabot. Dr. Cabot believed that children and adolescents develop behavior problems because they lack prosocial role models in their lives. He believed that at-risk youths could be "steered away from delinquency if a devoted individual outside his own family gives him consistent emotional support, friendship, and guidance" (McCord, 2010, p. 33).

To test this hypothesis, researchers recruited over 500 boys from Cambridge and Somerville, two densely populated, low-income neighborhoods near Boston. Many of the boys were identified by teachers as exhibiting conduct problems. At-risk boys without behavior problems were also recruited for the study to prevent stigma associated with participation.

The researchers matched boys based on certain characteristics that might predict their likelihood of delinquency, such as their intelligence, level of aggression, home environment, and parents' use of discipline. Then, the researchers randomly assigned one boy from each pair to a treatment group and the other boy to a control group.

Each boy in the treatment group was assigned a social worker who served as his mentor. Mentors met with each boy approximately twice every month: helping him with his homework, taking him to the YMCA or other activities, assisting him in finding a job, or engaging in sports or games. Mentors also worked with boys'

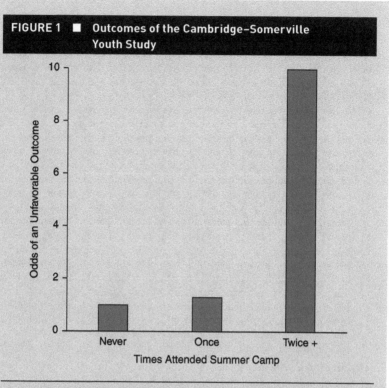

FIGURE 1 ■ Outcomes of the Cambridge–Somerville Youth Study

Note: Although therapeutic summer camps were designed to help at-risk youths, boys who attended these camps multiple times were more likely than other boys to have unfavorable outcomes later in life (Dishion et al., 1999).

families to help them improve the quality of family life. Boys in the treatment group were also allowed to attend a free summer camp with other boys in the program.

Boys in the control group received no special assistance, although they could seek treatment as usual in the community. The Cambridge-Somerville Youth Study lasted 5 years and was the first large-scale randomized controlled study investigating the effects of a psychosocial intervention on children.

Initial results were disappointing. Despite 5 years of mentoring, boys in the treatment group did not show better outcomes than the controls. Nevertheless, researchers remained optimistic that boys who received the treatment would fare better as adults.

Thirty years later, Joan McCord examined the long-term effects of the program. Amazingly, she was able to track down 98% of the boys who participated in the study. (They were now middle-aged men.) Then, she analyzed public databases, hospital logs, and court records to examine the boys' long-term outcomes.

(Continued)

[Continued]

Most of the boys who participated in the treatment recalled the program favorably. Similarly, most mentors believed that treatment had a positive impact on the boys' lives. However, when McCord examined the objective data, she was shocked. "It was so surprising," she said. "Everything was going in the wrong direction" (Zane, Welsh, & Zimmerman, 2017, p. 152).

McCord discovered that boys who received mentoring were more likely than controls to commit a felony, to develop substance use problems, or to manifest serious mental illness. Boys in the treatment group were also more likely than controls to have stress-related health problems, to report low job satisfaction, or to die at an earlier age. Indeed, 42% of boys who received mentoring experienced at least one of these "undesirable outcomes" compared to 32% of boys in the control group. The Cambridge-Somerville Youth Study backfired; it *increased* the likelihood of behavior problems in children who received treatment. What went wrong?

McCord and colleagues discovered that boys who spent more unstructured time with other boys in the program were at greatest risk for having negative outcomes later in life. In particular, boys who attended summer camp once during the treatment program were only 1.3 times more likely than controls to develop conduct problems. In contrast, attending camp multiple times increased a boy's likelihood of developing conduct problems 10-fold (Figure 1). The researchers concluded that boys talked about and reinforced each other's delinquent behavior during camp. The more time they spent at camp, the greater their likelihood of antisocial behavior later in life (Dishion, McCord, & Poulin, 1999).

Discussion Questions

1. How does the Cambridge-Somerville Youth Study illustrate the scientific principle of critical thinking?

2. Which of the four goals of psychological research did the Cambridge-Somerville Youth Study try to achieve?

3. Was the Cambridge-Somerville Youth Study's design cross-sectional or longitudinal?

4. The researchers discovered that the effects of treatment on children's outcomes depended on how many times they attended the summer camp. Boys who did not attend or attended the camp 1 time usually did not show undesirable outcomes, whereas boys who attended 2 or more times were at greater risk for undesirable outcomes. In this study, does "summer camp attendance" serve as a mediator or moderator variable?

5. What is the difference between random selection and random assignment? Which did the researchers use in the Cambridge-Somerville Youth Study?

6. What were the independent and dependent variables in the Cambridge-Somerville Youth Study?

7. What type of control group did the researchers use? What was one potential benefit of this type of control group?

8. What is attrition? How can it threaten the internal validity of a study? Was it a problem in the Cambridge-Somerville Youth Study?

9. What is external validity? In what way is the external validity of the Cambridge-Somerville Youth Study limited?

10. What can the Cambridge-Somerville Youth Study teach us about the causes of children's disorders?

11. What can the Cambridge-Somerville Youth Study teach us about the importance of psychological research, especially regarding the treatment of child and adolescent problems?

References

Dishion, T. J., McCord, J., & Poulin, F. (1999). When interventions harm. *American Psychologist, 54*, 755–764.

McCord, J. (2010). The Cambridge-Somerville study. In G. Sayre-McCord (Ed.), *Crime and family* (pp. 32–40). Philadelphia, PA: Temple University Press.

Zane, S. N., Welsh, B. C., & Zimmerman, G. M. (2017). Examining the iatrogenic effects of the Cambridge-Somerville Youth Study. *British Journal of Criminology, 56*, 141–160.

This case study accompanies the textbook: Weis, R. (2021). *Introduction to abnormal child and adolescent psychology* (4th ed.). Thousand Oaks, CA: Sage. Answers appear in the online instructor resources. Visit **https://sagepub.com**.

4

ASSESSING AND TREATING CHILDREN'S PROBLEMS

CASE STUDY
FUNCTIONAL ANALYSIS OF CHILDREN'S BEHAVIOR

Functional analysis is an assessment method in which professionals identify the antecedents and consequences of children's behavior problems. For each of these scenarios, explain how you might perform a functional analysis of behavior. Specifically, answer the following questions:

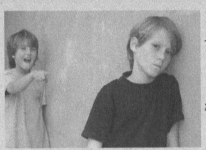

- How might you **operationally define** the behavior problem?

- What might be an **antecedent** of the behavior? How might this antecedent elicit the behavior?

- What might be a **consequence** of the behavior? How might this consequence reinforce the behavior and maintain it over time?

- How might you **intervene**, either by altering the antecedent or consequence of the behavior?

1. You are a psychologist working in an elementary school. You have been asked by one of the teachers at the school to deal with a fifth-grade student

who bullies other children. The teacher says the child's behavior is getting worse and she is growing very frustrated with him.

2. You are a therapist assigned to work with an extremely shy 7-year-old girl. She refuses to go to school because she fears criticism from her teacher and classmates. She has no friends and only seems comfortable at home.

3. Your client is a 34-year-old woman with a disrespectful son. The boy never does what she says, deliberately defies her, throws tantrums, and ignores her commands. She reports considerable stress in her role as a mother. She loves her son but doesn't enjoy spending time with him.

4. Your client is an 8-year-old boy with autism spectrum disorder and below-average intellectual functioning. He attends a regular second-grade classroom with help from an aide. Several times each hour, the boy engages in stereotypies: rocking back and forth and flapping his arms. His stereotyped behaviors are disruptive and distract his classmates during lessons.

5. Your teenage client reports problems with depression that have lasted approximately 4 months. She feels sad and lethargic most of the time, has dropped out of her favorite activities like the school pep and jazz bands, has a hard time getting out of bed in the morning, and can't concentrate on her schoolwork. She wants antidepressant medication and is furious when she finds out that you can't prescribe it because you're a psychologist and not a "real doctor."

6. You are a family therapist. One of your clients is a couple who has been married for 6 years. They have two young children. The wife complains that her husband doesn't listen to her or appreciate her. The husband complains that his wife is emotionally distant and frigid. They each say that the other one is argumentative. They are seeing you as a last-ditch effort before divorce.

This case study accompanies the textbook: Weis, R. (2021). *Introduction to abnormal child and adolescent psychology* (4th ed.). Thousand Oaks, CA: Sage. Answers appear in the online instructor resources. Visit **https://sagepub.com**.

CASE STUDY
WHAT MAKES A GOOD PSYCHOLOGICAL TEST?

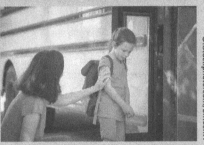

©iStockphoto.com/bmcent1

The Screen for Child Anxiety Related Emotional Disorders (SCARED) is one of the most widely used and well-validated measures of anxiety for children and adolescents (Birmaher et al., 1997). The current version of the SCARED is a questionnaire that assesses all of the major DSM-5 anxiety disorders, obsessive–compulsive disorder, posttraumatic stress disorder, and school refusal (Bodden, Bögels, & Muris, 2009). It can be administered to parents or youths aged 8 to 18 years. Here are some sample items (and the disorder they measure):

- When frightened, I feel dizzy . . . (panic disorder)
- I worry about the future . . . (generalized anxiety disorder)
- I don't like being away from my family . . . (separation anxiety disorder)
- It's hard for me to talk with people I don't know . . . (social phobia)
- I'm scared to go to school . . . (school refusal)

Let's imagine that it's 1997 and we have been asked to evaluate the reliability and validity of the SCARED. The Spice Girls and Backstreet Boys are playing on a CD in the background and we're ready to get to work!

Discussion Questions

1. The developers of the SCARED wanted to create a brief *questionnaire* that might identify children at risk for anxiety and related disorders. At that time, there were already several structured *interviews* that clinicians could use to identify anxiety disorders in children. Why did the researchers want to create a questionnaire, too?

2. The SCARED is a questionnaire that can be administered to both parents and children separately. Why was it important for the test's authors to develop a screening instrument that could be administered to both adults and children?

3. The SCARED is a norm-referenced test. What does it mean when we say that a test is "norm-referenced?" If we wanted to create the SCARED as a norm-referenced test, what would we need to do?

4. How might we assess the test-retest reliability of the SCARED?

5. How might we assess the internal consistency of the SCARED?

6. What is validity? Can a test be valid without being reliable?

7. How might we assess the content validity of the SCARED?

8. How might we assess the construct validity of the SCARED?

9. How might we assess the criterion-related validity of the SCARED?

References

Birmaher, B., Khetarpal, S., Brent, D., Cully, M., Balach, L., Kaufman, J., & Neer, S. M. (1997). The Screen for Child Anxiety Related Emotional Disorders (SCARED): Scale construction and psychometric characteristics. *Journal of the American Academy of Child and Adolescent Psychiatry, 36,* 545–553.

Bodden, D. H., Bögels, S. M., & Muris, P. (2009). The diagnostic utility of the Screen for Child Anxiety Related Emotional Disorders-71 (SCARED-71). *Behavior Research and Therapy, 47,* 418–425.

CASE STUDY

VAL REVISED: APPLYING THE SYSTEMS OF PSYCHOTHERAPY

There are hundreds of different systems or "schools" of psychotherapy. Chapter 4 in the text presents five broad approaches to therapy that are most often used with children and adolescents.

Let's look at the case of Val once again, the adolescent with an opioid use

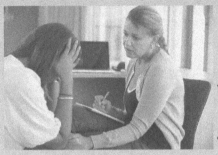

©iStockphoto.com/ monkeybusinessimages

disorder. If you were Val's therapist, what approach to treatment would you recommend? If you were Val, what approach to treatment would you prefer?

Description

Valerie Connell was a 16-year-old girl who was referred to an inpatient residential treatment program for adolescents with substance use disorders. Val was ordered to participate in treatment by the juvenile court after she was arrested for opioid possession and distribution.

Val grew up in a western suburb of Chicago. Her father was a musician with a history of alcohol and marijuana use problems. He left Val and her mother when Val was 5 years old. Although he continued to live in the Chicago area, he had only occasional contact with Val. Val had mixed feelings about her father. On one hand, she was attracted to his glamorous lifestyle: performing, traveling, and socializing. On the other hand, she resented his decision to abandon his family when she was so young and harbored anger toward him because of the many times he disappointed her over the years. "If your own dad doesn't care about you, no one will," said Val. "I saw myself as pretty worthless—like no one will ever really love me."

Val's mother also had a history of alcohol use. She became pregnant with Val when she was 17, a single parent by the time she was 22, and a recovering alcoholic by the time she was 26. Mrs. Connell attends Alcoholics Anonymous meetings to maintain her sobriety and supports herself and Val by working two jobs. Long hours limit her ability to be involved in Val's school or extracurricular activities. Although she says, "Val means the world to me—the one thing I live for," she admits that stress at work and concerns about her ability to pay the bills "sometimes cause me to lose my temper with her."

Val exhibited problems with hyperactivity and oppositional behavior as a preschooler. "She was a handful," recalled her mother. "She'd always be on the go, she never wanted to be quiet and listen to me. If I would tell her to do something, she'd ignore me, yell, or scream." Val's disruptive behavior persisted into elementary school. Her pediatrician prescribed stimulant medication to manage her hyperactive-impulsive behavior, but it had little effect on her defiance and tantrums. By the time Val was in the third grade, she was behind her classmates in reading and math and had gained a reputation as a troublemaker.

Val's substance use began with her transition to middle school. She was referred to a special education program for children with behavior problems and learning disabilities. She quickly made friends with several girls who introduced her to smoking (age 12) and marijuana (age 13). Although she tried alcohol at approximately the same age, she did not like its taste and limited its use to parties and social gatherings. By the time Val was 14 years old, she was using marijuana several times per week and drinking five to six sweet alcoholic drinks at parties on the weekends. She found it easy to hide her substance use from her mother.

Val transitioned to an alternative high school during her freshman year. "All of the kids there used drugs," Val recalled. Her 17-year-old boyfriend introduced her to prescription pain medication. Val's favorite combination was OxyContin in the morning followed by Roxicodone periodically throughout the school day. She quickly became known as the "Oxy and Roxy" girl. "I'd sleep during class, slur my speech, didn't care about anything," she recalled. "The teachers didn't say anything to me because I didn't cause trouble, so I kept on going." Val obtained $10 pills from her boyfriend and sold them to classmates for $25, pocketing the profits to support her own drug use.

"I first used heroin with my boyfriend—a different boyfriend—during my sophomore year," Val reported. "I was afraid of needles so I snorted it. The feeling was excellent, like all the pain in my life was taken away. I could relax, stay still, and not worry about school or family. Snorting worked much faster than taking pills and the effects of heroin were much better." Within 6 months, Val was using heroin approximately 3 times per day to sustain its positive effects and avoid withdrawal symptoms such as anxiety, nausea, and agitation. Her use became expensive and she engaged in prostitution several times to support her habit.

"It might seem crazy, but I'm kind of glad that I got caught," Val reported. "I've been to the funerals of two friends who died from heroin. My life was on the wrong track." In residential treatment, Val was prescribed a medication called Suboxone, a combination of buprenorphine (an opiate substitute that reduces cravings) and naloxone (a medication that blocks the positive effects of heroin). The physician and psychologist at the residential treatment facility hope that it will help her reduce her opioid use (see Fiellin et al., 2014).

"I'm not sure what I'm going to do when I get out of here," reported Val. "My mom wants me to come back home, but I can't go back. Everyone I know uses. I need a clean break."

Discussion Questions

1. According to Carl Rogers, what three necessary and sufficient factors might the therapist provide to help Val overcome her substance use problems.

2. How might a behavior therapist attempt to help Val with her opioid use disorder?

(Continued)

[Continued]

3. How might a cognitive therapist attempt to help Val with her opioid use disorder?

4. How might an interpersonal therapist attempt to help Val with her opioid use disorder?

5. How might a family systems therapist attempt to help Val with her opioid use disorder?

6. How might a psychodynamic therapist attempt to help Val with her opioid use disorder?

Reference

Fiellin, D. A., Schottenfeld, R. S., Cutter, C. J., Moore, B. A., Barry, D. T., & O'Connor, P. G. (2014). Primary care–based buprenorphine taper vs maintenance therapy for prescription opioid dependence: A randomized clinical trial. *JAMA Internal Medicine, 174*(12), 1947–1954.

This case study accompanies the textbook: Weis, R. (2021). *Introduction to abnormal child and adolescent psychology* (4th ed.). Thousand Oaks, CA: Sage. Answers appear in the online instructor resources. Visit **https://sagepub.com**. This case is based on interviews conducted by Paul Grondahl for the *Albany Times Union*.

CASE STUDIES OF CHILDREN AND ADOLESCENTS

5

INTELLECTUAL DISABILITY AND DEVELOPMENTAL DISORDERS

CASE STUDY

CHEERFUL ROBIN

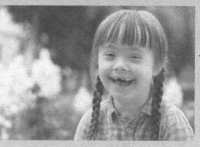

Milena was a 6-year-old girl who was referred to a school psychologist by her pediatrician. Milena was diagnosed with Down syndrome when she was an infant. Her pediatrician wanted Milena's cognitive and academic achievement skills to be reassessed before Milena started kindergarten in autumn.

Milena's gestation and delivery were uncomplicated. However, Milena was born with a congenital heart defect that required several surgeries. Milena showed physical features associated with Down syndrome. For example, she had a small nose with a flat nasal bridge, almond-shaped eyes, and broad hands with short

(Continued)

(Continued)

fingers. Each of her palms had a single transverse crease rather than the many folds seen in most children.

Milena showed delays in achieving developmental milestones, especially in the areas of gross motor functioning (e.g., sitting up, walking), fine motor skills (e.g., feeding and dressing herself), and expressive communication (e.g., saying her first words, using two- or three-word phrases). Fortunately, Milena's parents became active in her education and in a local support group for the caregivers of children with Down syndrome. Milena participated in occupational therapy and speech-language therapy as a toddler and attended a full-day enrichment preschool for children with special needs.

Results of the Wechsler Intelligence Scale for Children–Fifth Edition (WISC-V) indicated that Milena's full scale IQ (FSIQ) was 57, falling in the low range of intellectual functioning. Milena performed better on tests assessing her visual-spatial reasoning and nonverbal fluid reasoning than tests assessing her verbal comprehension skills. Her preschool teacher said that Milena often learned better through demonstrations and "hands-on" learning than from verbal instruction.

Milena showed good eye contact when speaking with others, obeyed classroom rules, and enjoyed playing with other children. With extensive practice, she also learned to perform self-care skills such as bathing, dressing, and cleaning her room. On the other hand, Milena continued to show problems learning her numbers, the alphabet, and the value of money. Her reading skills were poor and her handwriting was mostly illegible.

Interpersonally, Milena presented as a charming girl who loved to play with her classmates and spend time with her parents. Her favorite hobbies included playing soccer, petting her dog, and helping her parents cook meals. Her parents called her "the cheerful robin" because of her tendency to get up early in the morning and her friendly, social disposition.

Discussion Questions

1. List the three DSM-5 domains of adaptive functioning. Then, describe Milena's functioning on each of these three domains.

2. DSM-5 identifies four levels of severity for children with intellectual disability. Which level of severity best describes Milena's functioning?

3. According to Zigler's classification system, what is the difference between organic and cultural-familial intellectual disability? Which classification best describes youths with Down syndrome like Milena?

4. How do Milena's delays in gross motor, fine motor, and communication skills support the similar sequence hypothesis?

5. What is the behavioral phenotype for children with Down syndrome? How many aspects of this phenotype does Milena show?

6. What caused Milena's disability? Did she inherit Down syndrome from her parents?

7. What prenatal tests might Milena's mother have taken to determine the risk that Milena would be born with Down syndrome? Which of these tests carries the greatest risk to the fetus?

8. Milena's school psychologist would likely use the results of her assessment to generate an IEP for Milena. What is an IEP?

9. If you were Milena's teacher, how might you use principles of universal design to help Milena read and perform mathematics?

10. In what way might having a child with a known genetic disorder, like Down syndrome, be easier than having a child with a developmental disability of unknown origin?

This case study accompanies the textbook: Weis, R. (2021). *Introduction to abnormal child and adolescent psychology* (4th ed.). Thousand Oaks, CA: Sage. Answers appear in the online instructor resources. Visit **https://sagepub.com**.

CASE STUDY
NEW CHALLENGES

Logan was a 7-year-old boy referred to our clinic by his mother because of problems with hyperactivity and stereotyped behaviors at home and school. Logan was diagnosed with Fragile X syndrome at the age of 3½ years and attended a special-needs preschool for children with neurodevelopmental disorders. This year, Logan began first grade at his local public school and attends most regular classes with the help of a classroom aide.

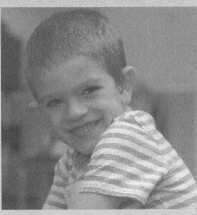

Image courtesy of Peter Saxon, Wikimedia Creative Commons

Logan reached developmental milestones at a much slower pace than other children his age. Most notably, he showed marked delays in fine and gross motor skills and generally poor muscle tone and coordination. He was very slow to develop receptive and expressive language and, even today, speaks in simple sentences. His speech is often perseverative and tangential; he often repeats words, phrases, and sounds. Logan was initially diagnosed with global developmental delay. Genetic testing later confirmed the existence of Fragile X.

Results of cognitive testing at the beginning of first grade showed that Logan's FSIQ was approximately 50. He showed relative strengths on tasks assessing visual-spatial processing and rote memory, but relative weaknesses on tasks measuring verbal abilities, abstract reasoning, and attention, even compared to other children at his developmental level.

Logan's mother was most concerned with his social behavior. Logan became easily excited in his new classroom. He had difficulty with transitions from one activity to the next, became anxious and overwhelmed during loud games or assemblies, and refused to participate in most group activities. Logan seldom made eye contact with teachers or peers. He seemed to want to make friends and to join groups, but he was extremely reticent to interact with others.

When anxious or excited, Logan would show signs of physiological arousal, like a flushed face and sweating. He would appear agitated and show hyperactive behavior, such as leaving his seat, pacing about the room, and repeating words and phrases. Logan also showed stereotypies at these times; usually, he would rock or sway his body and flap his hands repeatedly. On one occasion, Logan's teacher tried to calm him by holding him in his seat by his shoulders and talking with him gently. Her actions made Logan more agitated, however, and elicited a severe tantrum.

Logan's mother was also concerned about similar problems with hyperarousal and social anxiety at home. Besides his siblings, Logan has few friends in his neighborhood. His poor eye contact, reluctance to engage others, and stereotypies limit his mother's ability to participate in community activities with peers. Despite his interpersonal challenges, Logan's mother described him as a "loving and affectionate little guy who I cherish with all my heart."

Discussion Questions

1. Logan has Fragile X syndrome. Can he also be diagnosed with intellectual disability? If he meets diagnostic criteria for autism spectrum disorder (ASD), can he also be diagnosed with that condition, too?

2. Why was Logan diagnosed with global developmental delay as a toddler?

3. Logan displays stereotypies, especially when overaroused. What other challenging behaviors are sometimes shown by children with intellectual disability?

4. Do Logan's weaknesses in verbal abilities, abstract reasoning, and attention support the similar structure hypothesis?

5. What causes Fragile X syndrome?

6. Why are girls much less likely than boys to show Fragile X syndrome?

7. Imagine that you want to observe Logan's behavior at school in order to record the number of times he flaps his hands in a given class period. What method of observation might you use to record this frequency?

8. If you were Logan's parent or classroom aide, how might you use positive reinforcement to help him keep his hands at his side and reduce hand flapping?

9. Are any medications effective in reducing challenging behaviors in youths with developmental disabilities?

This case study accompanies the textbook: Weis, R. (2021). *Introduction to abnormal child and adolescent psychology* (4th ed.). Thousand Oaks, CA: Sage. Answers appear in the online instructor resources. Visit **https://sagepub.com**.

6

AUTISM SPECTRUM DISORDER

CASE STUDY

OUR MIRACLE

Joel was a 33-month-old boy referred to the developmental disabilities clinic of a large children's hospital. Joel's pediatrician had assigned a provisional diagnosis of autism spectrum disorder (ASD) and requested that the psychologists at the clinic perform a more thorough assessment and determine the best avenue for treatment.

Joel was born premature, weighing only 3½ pounds upon delivery. Moreover, he was diagnosed with neonatal anemia shortly after birth, a condition that limited the amount of oxygen in his bloodstream. He spent the first 6 weeks in and out of the hospital. His parents called him "our miracle" when he finally was deemed healthy enough to come home.

©iStockphoto.com/jarenwicklund

Joel was diagnosed with global developmental delay 18 months ago when he displayed marked delays in gross motor skills, fine motor skills, and language. His pediatrician attributed these early delays to his perinatal medical problems.

Today, however, Joel is largely unable to feed, dress, or otherwise care for himself, and he has limited receptive language skills and no functional expressive language. Joel also shows very little shared attention, rarely initiates interactions with other people besides his parents, and does not engage in pretend or symbolic play. Indeed, Joel seldom maintains eye contact with others and shows little interest in games or activities enjoyed by most children his age. Although Joel has many toys, his favorite pastimes are arranging and rearranging common household objects, dropping items onto the floor from his chair and noticing the sounds they make, and listening to music. His parents reported that he would engage in these activities "all day long" if they would let him.

"We've tried to improve Joel's self-care skills and use of language, but it's been very difficult," admitted his father. "When we make him use a spoon to eat, or require him to look us in the eye, he cries terribly. We know it's in his interest in the long term to do these things but he fights us every time, so we eventually just give in and let him do things his way."

Joel's mother added, "On a few occasions, he's become very upset. When we first started to brush his teeth, he would cry. Now, he tries to hit or bite us. We need help teaching him some skills so that he can go to school on his own."

The psychologist at the clinic attempted to assess Joel's intellectual functioning, but he refused to participate in testing. Results of the Autism Diagnostic Interview-Revised and the Autism Diagnostic Observation Schedule, Second Edition confirmed Joel's diagnosis of ASD.

"We're hoping that you can help us obtain services from our school district," Joel's father said to the psychologist. "We also need help improving his behavior at home."

Discussion Questions

1. List four problem areas or deficits shown by Joel.

2. Which problem areas reflect his DSM-5 ASD diagnosis and which problem areas are associated with ASD but are *not* part of the diagnosis itself?

3. What deficits in social cognition did Joel show as a toddler that preceded his ASD diagnosis?

4. What evidence-based psychosocial treatments might you recommend for Joel to help improve his social communication and language skills?

5. If Joel is lucky enough to live in a community where the Treatment and Education of Autistic and Related Communication-Handicapped Children (TEACCH) approach is available, what might this intervention look like?

(Continued)

(Continued)

6. The psychologist at the clinic recommends that Joel's family use an augmentative and alternative communication (AAC) system to help Joel communicate. What is an AAC system? Will an AAC system limit Joel's use of verbal language?

7. When Joel's parents try to brush Joel's teeth, he cries and sometimes becomes aggressive. His parents back down and let him go without brushing his teeth. Over time, Joel learns that crying is an effective way to avoid activities he dislikes. In behavioral terms, what sort of reinforcement has occurred?

8. BONUS: In Chapter 5, we learned how to conduct a functional analysis of problem behavior in children with developmental disabilities. How might you use this method to determine the function of Joel's crying, hitting, and biting?

Reference

Iwata, B. A., Pace, G. M., Dorsey, M. F., Zarcone, J. R., Vollmer, T. R., Smith, R. G., . . . Goh, H. L. (1994). The functions of self injurious behavior: An experimental epidemiological analysis. *Journal of Applied Behavior Analysis, 27,* 215–240.

This case study accompanies the textbook: Weis, R. (2021). *Introduction to abnormal child and adolescent psychology* (4th ed.). Thousand Oaks, CA: Sage. Answers appear in the online instructor resources. Visit **https://sagepub.com**.

CASE STUDY
A SECOND OPINION

Noah Favero was a 9-year-old boy referred to our clinic by his parents. Approximately 6 months ago, Noah's pediatrician diagnosed him with attention-deficit/hyperactivity disorder (ADHD) and began prescribing stimulant medication to help manage episodes of hyperactivity and impulsivity at school. Noah's parents reported that the medication was largely ineffective in reducing these episodes and they felt that "ADHD" did not adequately reflect Noah's behavior.

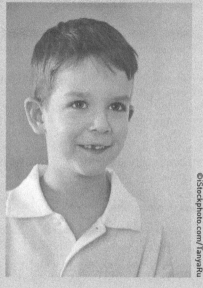

©iStockphoto.com/TanyaRu

Noah was a full-term, healthy infant who met early developmental milestones in an age-expected fashion. His parents began having concerns about his development at age 18 months, when Noah still did not show any spoken language. Also, Noah did not seem to interact with his parents like other toddlers his age. For example, he was content to play with toy trains and dinosaurs, lining them up and then rearranging them, for hours at a time. He seldom engaged his parents in play and rarely (if ever) engaged in pretend play with his toys. Noah also showed little interest in imitative games like "peekaboo" and "the itsy-bitsy spider." His parents attributed these behaviors to the fact that Noah was a "late bloomer."

Noah's expressive vocabulary developed rapidly between 30 and 36 months. By age 4, Noah was a talkative preschooler. His speech was characterized by two peculiarities, however. First, it had an odd, pedantic quality, as if Noah was lecturing *to* others rather than talking *with* others. Second, Noah was preoccupied with reptiles. Although such a fascination is not uncommon for a 4-year-old boy, Noah could not deviate from the subject. He exhausted his parents, relatives, and neighbors with information about lizards, snakes, and turtles.

Noah's behavior became more problematic when he began preschool. He seldom initiated interactions with other children, except to talk about his favorite topic. He avoided group games and activities, especially when they were unstructured. Instead, Noah preferred to watch other children from the sidelines or to play by himself. Needless to say, Noah had few friends in preschool or in his neighborhood. Moreover, he did not seem bothered by his social isolation or aware of the fact that his behavior caused classmates to avoid him.

(Continued)

(Continued)

Noah displayed episodes of hyperactivity at school. His teacher reported that he would easily become overwhelmed by noisy activities and transitions from one class to the next. During these instances, he would pace about the classroom, talk incessantly, or rock in his seat. More concerning, Noah would become irritable or angry when forced to engage in certain high-rate group activities. During one class assembly, for example, he yelled and threw a chair when he was asked to accompany his class to sing onstage. On another occasion, Noah became belligerent when his daily schedule was changed to accommodate a Halloween party.

On the WISC-V, Noah earned a FSIQ in the average range. He showed above-average scores on measures of verbal comprehension and visual-spatial reasoning, but below-average scores on measures of working memory and processing speed. His reading, writing, and math skills were within the average range.

"We're hoping that you might be able to give us a second opinion about Noah," said his father. "The school psychologist recommended that we have him evaluated more thoroughly." Noah's mother added, "She said that many of his behaviors resemble the features of autism, but that doesn't seem right."

Discussion Questions

1. Review the DSM-5 diagnostic criteria for ASD. Which features does Noah display?

2. Can Noah be diagnosed with ASD despite the fact that his FSIQ is within the average range and he has good verbal skills?

3. How does Noah display problems with the pragmatics of language?

4. Many toddlers later diagnosed with ASD show early deficits in social communication. What deficits did Noah show as a toddler?

5. Why might early intensive behavioral intervention (EIBI) probably *not* be the first-line treatment for Noah? If you were Noah's therapist, what skills would you target for treatment?

6. BONUS: Although some youths with ASD also have ADHD, Noah's behavior does *not* support the existence of comorbid ADHD. Why not?

This case study accompanies the textbook: Weis, R. (2021). *Introduction to abnormal child and adolescent psychology* (4th ed.). Thousand Oaks, CA: Sage. Answers appear in the online instructor resources. Visit **https://sagepub.com**.

7

COMMUNICATION AND LEARNING DISORDERS

CASE STUDY

ANIMAL NOISES

Josie is a 24-month-old girl who shows speech and language problems. Josie's parents brought her to you, her pediatrician.

"Josie's vocabulary seems very underdeveloped," her mother reported. "She doesn't know very many words. She can make the correct noises for several animals when she sees them in a picture book, but she doesn't know the names of any of the animals."

Her father added, "Josie also doesn't seem to understand simple questions, like 'Do you want juice?' or obey simple commands like, 'Give me your doll.'"

You quickly determine that Josie is physically healthy with vision and hearing within normal limits. She is able to point to her eyes and ears when you ask her to do so,

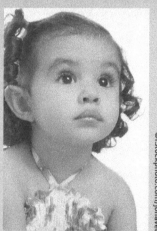

©iStockphoto.com/johavel

but she isn't able to follow more complex, two-step commands (e.g., *get the ball and throw it into the basket*). Josie says "hi" and "bye" but is otherwise nonverbal. Her eye contact is ample during your assessment, and she seldom strays from her parents.

After the session, Josie's parents ask you, "So, do you think something is wrong with Josie? If so, what should we do about it?"

(Continued)

(Continued)

Discussion Questions

1. How would you assess Josie's language skills?

2. What DSM-5 diagnosis best describes Josie's communication problems?

3. What other (differential) diagnoses might you want to rule out?

4. What is Josie's prognosis?

5. How might you use discrete trial training to increase Josie's use of language?

This case study accompanies the textbook: Weis, R. (2021). *Introduction to abnormal child and adolescent psychology* (4th ed.). Thousand Oaks, CA: Sage. Answers appear in the online instructor resources. Visit **https://sagepub.com**.

CASE STUDY
PRODUCTION PROBLEMS

You are a speech-language therapist at a local elementary school. One of the kindergarten teachers at your school referred her student to you, a 6-year-old boy named Jack. Jack had a history of language delays as a preschooler and had received speech therapy for problems with articulation prior to beginning school. Currently, his language skills are still poor.

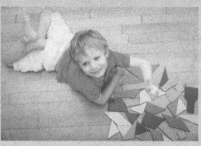

"I can't understand what Jack is saying most of the time," his teacher reported. "He often says 'gar' for *car* and 'gook' for *book*. Jack often makes simple mistakes when speaking. For example, today he said, 'Me got two gars' instead of *I have two cars.* Yesterday, he described a classmate running in the hallway, saying, 'Him run in gall.' In general, Jack talks like a 3-year-old rather than a boy his age."

You meet with Jack and briefly screen his receptive and expressive vocabulary. You notice that Jack has difficulty finding the right words to label objects. For example, when shown a picture of a watch, he called it a "tock" (i.e., clock). When shown a picture of a purse, he called it "Dat ting mom has. I not know what." You also discover that Jack's ability to recognize letters and word sounds (i.e., phonemes) is below average. For example, he was only able to correctly identify 14 letters and he was unable to generate the sounds for the letters f, l, and s.

"What should we do?" Jack's teacher asks.

Discussion Questions

1. What DSM-5 diagnosis best describes Jack's communication skills?

2. Describe Jack's phonology, morphology, grammar, and semantics.

3. Identify three possible causes for Jack's language problems.

4. How might you use conversational recast training to help Jack?

5. How might you use milieu training to help Jack?

This case study accompanies the textbook: Weis, R. (2021). *Introduction to abnormal child and adolescent psychology* (4th ed.). Thousand Oaks, CA: Sage. Answers appear in the online instructor resources. Visit **https://sagepub.com**.

CASE STUDY
SPEECH THERAPY

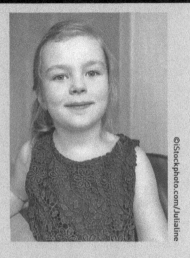

©iStockphoto.com/Juliaîine

Doria is a first-grade student who was referred to you because of problems with speech and language. As the speech-language therapist at the school, it is your job to assess Doria and to plan treatment, if you think it is appropriate.

Doria's main problem is speech production. Specifically, she has difficulty pronouncing the /r/ and /l/ phonemes. To informally assess her speech, you ask Doria what she likes to do on the weekends. She replies, "I weally wike to visit my dad. We wike to go to the movies or to the pawk."

You question Doria's mother about her speech problems. She replies, "Doria's been talking this way since the age of 2. She has a wonderful vocabulary and is very social. However, people have a hard time understanding her. They often ask her to repeat herself. Doria doesn't seem to mind too much."

Discussion Questions

1. What is Doria's primary DSM-5 diagnosis?

2. What is the chance that Doria will "grow out of" her speech problem? Does she need therapy?

3. Identify the most common reason for her speech problem.

4. How might a speech-language therapist provide speech therapy for Doria?

This case study accompanies the textbook: Weis, R. (2021). *Introduction to abnormal child and adolescent psychology* (4th ed.). Thousand Oaks, CA: Sage. Answers appear in the online instructor resources. Visit **https://sagepub.com**.

CASE STUDY

JUST BABY TALK?

You meet Geoffrey while volunteering at a local preschool. Geoffrey, a friendly 5-year-old boy, immediately likes you and wants to play. Although he is social and outgoing, Geoffrey's speech is poor. It is very difficult for you to understand Geoffrey and you frequently need to ask him to repeat himself. After talking with him for a while, you realize that he tends to omit or reverse the sounds in certain words. For example, when you ask him about his favorite games, he answers, "I lie do blay wi my drober. We blay babbetba by da hou." When you ask him about his favorite foods, he answers, "My pravite poods are mambergers, hotdas, an ide ream."

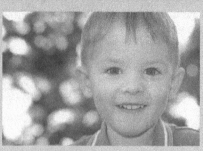
©iStockphoto.com/Sonsedska

You share your observations with Geoffrey's preschool teacher. She comments, "Geoffrey has always had articulation problems. He has excellent receptive vocabulary and knows what he wants to say. He is just very difficult to understand. Many kids his age have articulation problems or engage in baby talk. We are not too worried. His speech will improve when he starts first grade."

Discussion Questions

1. What DSM-5 diagnosis best describes Geoffrey's condition?

2. Identify one possible cause of his speech problem.

3. What is Geoffrey's prognosis? Will he improve without therapy?

4. If you were a speech-language therapist, how might you help Geoffrey?

This case study accompanies the textbook: Weis, R. (2021). *Introduction to abnormal child and adolescent psychology* (4th ed.). Thousand Oaks, CA: Sage. Answers appear in the online instructor resources. Visit **https://sagepub.com**.

CASE STUDY
TEASED IN SCHOOL

Mark is a 9-year-old boy enrolled in the fourth grade at a local elementary school. Several years ago, Mark began stuttering.

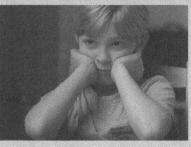

©iStockphoto.com/ KatarzynaBialasiewicz

"Mark began repeating certain letter sounds and syllables," his mother recalled. "It was amazing how quickly the problem began. Over the course of a few weeks, it became very noticeable. He would have trouble spitting words out. He would take long pauses, like he knew what he wanted to say, but couldn't actually articulate the words." She added, "Then, we noticed that he would tense up or grimace a little while trying to find the word he wanted. This became very noticeable to everyone. I think other kids teased him about it."

With his mother present, you interview Mark in order to get a sample of his speech. When asked to talk about school, Mark said, "I-I-I-I reall-lly like school. I-I-I-I lllll-ike art and mmm-usic the b-b-b-est. Ssss-."

His mother interrupted, "Don't worry honey. Take your time."

Mark continued, "Ssss-sometimes I have a hard ttt-ime in rrrrr-eading in class."

After Mark left the room, his mother added, "Mark's dad stuttered as a kid. He doesn't stutter now. We're hoping that Mark will outgrow this problem. What do you think?"

Discussion Questions

1. What is the official DSM-5 diagnosis for problems associated with stuttering?

2. What is the evidence that stuttering is heritable?

3. What brain differences are observable in children who do and do not stutter?

4. How might learning theory, emotion theory, and psycholinguistic theory be used to explain the causes of stuttering?

5. What is the likelihood that Mark will overcome his stuttering problem on his own?

6. How might a therapist improve Mark's speech?

This case study accompanies the textbook: Weis, R. (2021). *Introduction to abnormal child and adolescent psychology* (4th ed.). Thousand Oaks, CA: Sage. Answers appear in the online instructor resources. Visit **https://sagepub.com**.

CASE STUDY
PROBLEMS MAKING FRIENDS

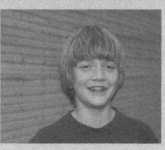

©iStockphoto.com/spfoto

Thirteen-year-old Ethan was referred by his parents, who were concerned with his social functioning. His father explained, "I asked to meet with you because you are the psychologist at Ethan's school. Ethan's a great kid. He's really bright and musically gifted. He does well in school and especially likes art, math, and science. All the time, he tells me how much he wants to be an engineer, like me, and work for my company when he grows up. But Ethan has problems making friends. He really wants friends and he's invited several kids over to the house. But he doesn't seem to know how to play with the other kids. For example, when other kids are playing a game, Ethan doesn't know how to join in. Then, if he sometimes manages to join the game, he insists on directing everything—being in charge."

Ethan's mother added, "He's also pretty pedantic. He goes on and on about topics no other kid really cares about. I think it turns them off or wears them out over time. Kids come to the house to play maybe once or twice but they seldom return."

You agree to meet with Ethan in your office the following day. With an awkward gait, Ethan enters your office, sits down on your chair, and comments, "You would have really enjoyed it."

"Enjoyed what?" you ask.

Ethan responds, "My little brother and I loved it, but my mom said it was too violent. I knew you would have loved it because you like those kinds of things and because you're young, not like my mom and dad. You don't look old enough to have read the original *Marvel* comics but you probably read the newer version when you were in school." Ethan looks over at the *Guardians of the Galaxy* figurine on your desk.

"Do you mean that I would have liked the *Guardians of the Galaxy* movie?" you ask. "I saw it. I liked it a lot. What did you like about it?"

Ethan replies, "The original *Marvel* comics came out when my dad was a kid—about my age. Things were a lot different back then. Rocket had a different name."

You ask, "They had rockets in the original?"

Ethan replies in a disgusted tone, "I thought you said you saw the movie? Not 'rockets.' I mean 'Rocket' the raccoon."

"Oh, right. I forgot his name until you mentioned it," you respond. "My favorite character was actually Groot, the plant-man. Did you think he was funny?"

Ethan replies, "Then, maybe 20 years passed before they resurrected the series and produced the new comics. Most people say that the original was better but I like the newer ones. . . . "

(Continued)

(Continued)

Discussion Questions

1. What DSM-5 communication disorder best describes Ethan's behavior?

2. What other (differential) diagnoses might you want to rule out?

3. How might you encourage Ethan to show better turn-taking skills?

4. What is conversational repair and how might you improve Ethan's conversational repair skills?

5. What are narratives and how might you improve Ethan's narrative skills?

This case study accompanies the textbook: Weis, R. (2021). *Introduction to abnormal child and adolescent psychology* (4th ed.). Thousand Oaks, CA: Sage. Answers appear in the online instructor resources. Visit **https://sagepub.com**.

CASE STUDY
DELAYS OR DEFICITS?

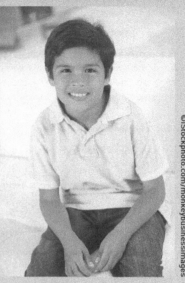

©iStockphoto.com/monkeybusinessimages

Sebastián is a 9-year-old, third-grade student referred to you for a psychological evaluation to determine whether he has a learning disability and might qualify for special education services. Information about Sebastián's early development is limited. His parents, both migrant workers, moved to the United States when Sebastián was a toddler. His mother and father speak Spanish exclusively at home and have limited English-speaking skills. Sebastián acquired English during his preschool years through his interactions with other children, involvement in his church, summer programs for the children of migrant workers, and 1 year of formal kindergarten. A recent physical exam indicated that he is healthy and has no vision or hearing problems.

Sebastián began showing delays in reading acquisition when he enrolled in his current school as a first-grade student. Although his receptive and expressive vocabulary were similar to other children his age, Sebastián could recognize only 16 of his letters and lacked the ability to phonetically decode (i.e., "sound out") letter combinations (such as *th*, *st*, *tr*) or simple words (such as *fish*, *pet*, *stop*). The COVID-19 pandemic caused Sebastián to miss a lot of school later that academic year. Consequently, his teacher was uncertain whether his reading delays were attributable to missed learning opportunities at school, his history of impoverished educational opportunities, the fact that English is his second language, or an underlying learning disability.

In second grade, Sebastián's reading skills fell further behind his classmates. Curriculum-based assessment using the Dynamic Indicators of Basic Early Literacy Skills (DIBELS) indicated the need for additional tutoring. Consequently, Sebastián progressed through Tier I and II interventions of the school's response to intervention (RTI) program. Although he showed some improvement in response to Tier II, small-group instruction, his reading skills continued to lag behind his peers at the end of second grade.

You decide to conduct a comprehensive assessment of Sebastián's cognitive and academic functioning. Because his English-speaking skills are excellent, you administer the English versions of all tests. On the WISC-V, Sebastián earned an FSIQ of 103, squarely within the average range. His verbal comprehension score

(Continued)

(Continued)

was slightly lower than his fluid and visual-spatial reasoning scores, but all three scores were within normal limits. Sebastián earned a score of 82 in processing speed, indicating below-average ability to process information quickly and easily.

On the Woodcock-Johnson IV Tests of Achievement (WJ-IV), Sebastián's Broad Math score of 101 fell within the average range. However, his performance on the Broad Written Language (85) and Broad Reading (78) composites was below average compared to other children his age. In fact, Sebastián's Broad Reading score exceeded only 7% of children his age in the standardization sample. Follow-up testing indicated basic reading skills similar to those of a typically developing first-grade student.

Discussion Questions

1. Does Sebastián meet DSM-5 diagnostic criteria for a specific learning disorder?

2. How did Sebastián's teachers try to use RTI to identify and correct his early reading deficits?

3. What is the difference between curriculum-based assessment and norm-referenced assessment? Which type of assessment did Sebastián receive?

4. Are children whose primary language is not English at greater risk for learning disabilities than native English speakers?

5. What is phonemic mediation and why might it be important to explain Sebastián's reading problems?

6. What intervention has the greatest empirical support for children with reading deficits like Sebastián?

This case study accompanies the textbook: Weis, R. (2021). *Introduction to abnormal child and adolescent psychology* (4th ed.). Thousand Oaks, CA: Sage. Answers appear in the online instructor resources. Visit **https://sagepub.com**.

CASE STUDY
NOT ADDING UP

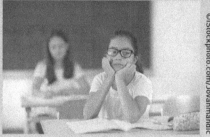

Maddie is an 11-year-old girl who was referred to you by her parents because of her recent decline in math performance at school.

"Maddie's a great kid. She's very conscientious, always tries her best, and loves to read and write," reported her father.

Her mother added, "She used to like math too. She learned to count, add, and subtract without much trouble. She started to struggle when she tried to learn multiplication. It took FOREVER for her to learn her times tables. I think she still has problems with some of them."

"Since that time, about third or fourth grade, Maddie has really struggled in math," said her father. "Initially, her teacher provided after-school tutoring for her. When that didn't work, she was placed in a special class for kids who had difficulty with math. We didn't notice much improvement, so we hired a tutor on our own. The tutor helps Maddie with her homework, but I'm not sure it has really helped her acquire the skills she needs."

You ask Maddie, "How do you feel about math?" With an embarrassed look, Maddie begins to speak, pauses, then starts to cry. "I hate it," eventually escapes from her mouth. "Nothing I do is ever right."

You decide to conduct a comprehensive evaluation to assess Maddie's intellectual abilities and academic achievement. Results of the WISC-V indicated an FSIQ of 115, above average compared to other children her age. Maddie's standard scores showed a significant strength in verbal comprehension (119) but a significant weakness in working memory (81). Follow-up testing confirmed that Maddie has marked deficits in both her verbal and nonverbal working memory compared to other youths her age.

As you expected, Maddie's reading and written language scores on the WJ-IV were well above average. Unfortunately, her score of 80 on the Broad Math domain was below average. Interestingly, Maddie earned an average score on a test of math fluency, indicating that she could solve simple arithmetic problems quickly and efficiently. However, her ability to perform higher-level math calculations and story problems was very delayed, exceeding only 5% of youths her age in the norm group.

Discussion Questions

1. Does Maddie meet DSM-5 diagnostic criteria for a specific learning disorder?

(Continued)

(Continued)

2. Maddie earned a very low score on the WISC-V working memory index. What is working memory and why might it be important to understand the cause of Maddie's problems with math?

3. Neither Maddie nor her parents reported problems with her reading skills. Why was it important to assess Maddie's reading skills when assessing her for a learning disability?

4. What three interventions are effective in helping students with math disabilities, like Maddie?

5. BONUS: How might Maddie's thoughts about math interfere with her ability to accurately solve math problems and do well in math class? If you were her parent, teacher, or therapist, how could you help Maddie think differently about math?

This case study accompanies the textbook: Weis, R. (2021). *Introduction to abnormal child and adolescent psychology* (4th ed.). Thousand Oaks, CA: Sage. Answers appear in the online instructor resources. Visit **https://sagepub.com**.

8

ATTENTION-DEFICIT/ HYPERACTIVITY DISORDER

CASE STUDY

LITTLE RED ROOSTER

Tricia Newsome slumped into the large chair in my office, looking much older than the 35 years she indicated on the new patient information sheet. "I'm at my wits' end," she began. "I'm coming to you because I don't know where else to go." With downcast eyes outlined by dark circles, she explained the reason for her visit: her 6-year-old son, Bennett.

Mr. and Mrs. Newsome were overjoyed when they discovered that they would finally have a child after many years of infertility. Mr. Newsome was an ecologist whose job allowed him to work outdoors most of the year, trapping, tagging, and monitoring animals

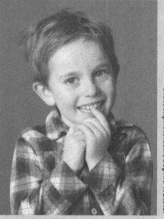

for the fish and wildlife service. Mrs. Newsome was a pharmaceutical representative who decided shortly after Bennett's birth to stay home with her newborn baby. The couple doted on Bennett who they described as a healthy, bouncing baby boy.

(Continued)

(Continued)

The problem, according to Mrs. Newsome, was that Bennett never stopped bouncing. "Even as an infant, Bennett was restless. He never wanted to eat and I had to force him to take a bottle. Later, when he began to eat solids, I had to fight to keep him in the high chair or at the table. He was also an erratic sleeper. He didn't sleep through the night until he was over 12 months of age—if you call sleeping 6 hours 'sleeping through the night.' Every morning, he'd wake up before sunrise and get into mischief. My husband called him 'the little red rooster' because of his early-morning waking, but I prayed that one day he might sleep later and let me rest."

"Bennett is a handful." Mrs. Newsome continued, "He's always moving—his legs, his arms, his middle. He can't sit still for more than a few minutes at a time and he has absolutely no attention span. He'll begin one activity, like playing with toy cars, and then move on to another activity after only a few minutes. My home is a mess because he leaves his toys everywhere."

Mrs. Newsome said, "Bennett's also a chatterbox. He never stops talking. It doesn't really matter if I'm listening or not; he'll even talk to himself. He'll interrupt me when I'm talking to other people, on the telephone, or doing work on the computer. He demands constant attention."

"Does Bennett act the same way at school?" I asked.

Mrs. Newsome replied, "That's why I'm here. His teacher wants me to take him to his pediatrician and get medication for ADHD. Apparently, Bennett engages in the same high-rate behavior at school as at home. He doesn't listen to directions, can't wait his turn, and frequently interrupts lessons. His classmates have started to avoid him because they find his behavior aversive."

I asked, "Is Bennett ever deliberately disrespectful to you or your husband? For example, does he talk back to you, refuse to do chores, or lose his temper?"

She replied, "Not any more than other first-graders. His teacher says that he tries hard to behave, but he can't help himself. It's as if he has more energy than most kids his age and doesn't know what to do with it."

Mrs. Newsome added, "Do you think Bennett has ADHD? He seems to have all of the features, according to WebMD. I really don't want to put him on medication. He's so young."

Discussion Questions

1. Review the DSM-5 signs and symptoms of ADHD. Which signs or symptoms does Bennett show, based on reports from his mother and teacher?

2. What DSM-5 diagnosis best describes Bennett's behavior, based on the available information?

3. Imagine that Bennett showed hyperactive-impulsive behavior only at home, but not at school. Could he still be diagnosed with ADHD? Why or why not?

4. Why did the psychologist ask Bennett's mother if Bennett was deliberately disrespectful to adults?

5. How common is it for a young child, like Bennett, to exhibit mostly hyperactive-impulsive symptoms, but not inattentive symptoms?

6. Why might the psychologist who conducted the evaluation want to assess Bennett's cognitive and academic skills?

7. How common are sleep problems among children with ADHD? Identify two sleep disorders typically shown by these children.

8. The psychologist did not ask whether Bennett's mother or father had problems with attention or hyperactivity-impulsivity as children or if they experience similar problems today. Why might assessing the family's history for ADHD be important?

9. Mrs. Newsome is reluctant to allow Bennett to take medication to manage his symptoms. What evidence-based, psychosocial treatments are available for children his age?

10. The psychologist wants Mrs. Newsome to make an informed decision regarding the best form of treatment for Bennett: medication, psychosocial treatment, or combined medication/psychosocial treatment. Based on the available empirical evidence, what should the psychologist tell her?

This case study accompanies the textbook: Weis, R. (2021). *Introduction to abnormal child and adolescent psychology* (4th ed.). Thousand Oaks, CA: Sage. Answers appear in the online instructor resources. Visit **https://sagepub.com**.

CASE STUDY
FORGOTTEN FAITH

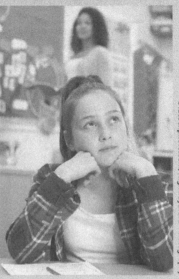

Eleven-year-old Faith sat in the front row of her fifth-grade classroom, listening to her teacher explain the difference between proper and common nouns. But Faith wasn't really listening. Anyone visiting her class that day would have thought that Faith was a model student. She sat at her desk quietly, eyes forward, feet solidly on the floor, chewing on the side of her pencil. Her teacher knew better.

"Faith," Mrs. Kline said, abruptly pausing the lesson. "Are you with us?"

Faith's eyes suddenly widened. She shook her head, oriented herself to her teacher, and glanced quickly around the room at her classmates who were beginning to snicker. Of course, Faith had no idea what the subject of today's lesson was. For at least the last 15 minutes, her mind had wandered from language arts, to crows outside her classroom window, to last night's soccer game, to a friend's upcoming birthday party, to whatever. Her teacher's reprimand brought Faith back to earth.

Faith began to show problems with inattention and mind wandering only in the past academic year. Mrs. Kline initially thought that Faith was sick or not getting sufficient sleep at home. She seemed to be chronically tired, slow, and lethargic. After Faith's parents (and pediatrician) confirmed that she was healthy, Mrs. Kline looked for other explanations for Faith's inattentiveness. Maybe she was depressed or preoccupied by troubles at home? Maybe she had a learning disability and had difficulty following lessons? Maybe she couldn't see the board?

Assessment by the school psychologist and nurse ruled out these possibilities. Moving Faith's desk to the front row of the classroom, periodically calling on her to direct her attention, and pasting sticky notes to her desk to remind her of important assignments did not help. Faith still couldn't focus on lessons, made careless mistakes on assignments and tests, and didn't complete activities that lasted for more than a few minutes. Her desk and locker were a mess because of her poor organizational skills.

As Mrs. Kline returned to her lesson, Faith's eyes gradually began to glaze over. She tried very hard to focus on which nouns need to be capitalized and which do not. She knew that information would be important for the test tomorrow. But, for some reason, it was no longer important. Faith's attention was now on the scarf in Mrs. Kline's hair. How had she not noticed it before? It had a butterfly pattern that resembled a monarch. She wondered if the milkweed would grow in the field near her house again this year, what other kinds of foods monarchs might eat if milk-weed was not available, and what she might eat for dinner tonight. . . .

Discussion Questions

1. What DSM-5 signs or symptoms of ADHD does Faith show?

2. What additional information would we need to know in order to diagnose Faith with ADHD, predominantly inattentive presentation?

3. What features of "sluggish cognitive tempo" does Faith display?

4. In samples of clinic-referred children, the gender ratio for ADHD favors boys, approximately 10:1. In samples of children from the community, the gender ratio is only 3:1. What might explain this difference?

5. What is the default mode network and why might it be important in explaining Faith's attention problems at school?

6. Can improving children's duration and/or quality of sleep reduce their inattentive symptoms?

This case study accompanies the textbook: Weis, R. (2021). *Introduction to abnormal child and adolescent psychology* (4th ed.). Thousand Oaks, CA: Sage. Answers appear in the online instructor resources. Visit **https://sagepub.com**.

9

CONDUCT PROBLEMS IN CHILDREN AND ADOLESCENTS

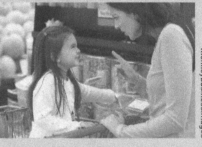

baby. I'm just getting a few things and then we're going home to bed," Amanda replied.

Jamie didn't like that answer. She repeated her request. Then, she began to complain, then whine, then cry. "I'm so hungry. Why can't I? Please???" Jamie kicked the shopping cart in time with her protests for added emphasis.

Amanda was sure that Jamie was acting this way deliberately to annoy her. Jamie knew how to press her buttons, especially at the end of the day. The check-out person, clearly perturbed, narrowed her eyes on Amanda. Amanda could read the checkout person's mind, "Don't you have any control over your kid? Why didn't you feed her a decent meal? What are you doing at the supermarket with a 5-year-old at 9:30 on a school-night in the first place?" Amanda felt a flood of emotions: anger, despair, fatigue.

Discussion Question

Gerald Patterson (2016) identified a problematic pattern of parent–child inter-actions known as coercive family process. Based on Patterson's research, how should Amanda respond to her daughter *and why*?

a. Buy Jamie the peanut bar. After all, peanuts are healthy, right?

b. Stand firm, even if that means yelling or threatening Jamie with punishment. You need to show her who's the parent and who's the child.

c. Ignore her. Let her protest all she wants. She might tantrum in the middle of the supermarket, but hey—it's Walmart. She won't be the first kid to do that.

References

Patterson, G. R. (2016). Coercion theory: The study of change. In T. J. Dishion & J. J. Snyder (Eds.), *Oxford handbook of coercive relationship dynamics* (pp. 7–22). Oxford, England: Oxford University Press.

This case study accompanies the textbook: Weis, R. (2021). *Introduction to abnormal child and adolescent psychology* (4th ed.). Thousand Oaks, CA: Sage. Answers appear in the online instructor resources. Visit **https://sagepub.com**.

CASE STUDY
SIDELINED!

Twelve-year-old Aiden loved soccer. That's why it was sheer torture for him to miss even a minute of recess. All morning long, he waited for the chance to escape his classroom and run to the field outside his school to play during lunchtime.

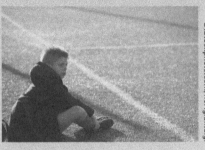

Unfortunately, today Aiden was late for recess because he had "lunch duty" and it was his responsibility to make sure the tables were clean after everyone had eaten. When he was finished, Aiden dashed to the soccer field. Dismayed, he discovered that the other boys had already started and were in the middle of a close game.

"Which team should I be on?" Aiden asked one of the boys.

The boy responded curtly, "Neither. Take a seat."

Another boy said, "Yeah. The game's too close." Several other boys snickered and then ran off after the ball.

Aiden felt a rush of warmth spread from the middle of his chest to the center of his face. He didn't know exactly how he felt. Was it pain? Disappointment? Rejection? Anger? Whatever the feeling, it was not good and Aiden knew he needed to do something about it.

Discussion Questions

1. Identify the six main components of Crick and Dodge's (1994, 1996) social information-processing model.

2. If Aiden was a boy with a history of reactive aggression, what sort of biases might he show in his social information processing?

3. If Aiden was a boy with a history of proactive aggression, what sort of biases might he show in his social information processing?

4. After Aiden enacts his solution to this social problem, how does the social information-processing model repeat itself?

5. If you were Aiden's therapist, how might you use problem-solving skills training (PSST) to help him avoid conflicts with peers?

References

Crick, N. R., & Dodge, K. A. (1994). A review and reformulation of social information-processing mechanisms in children's social adjustment. *Psychological Bulletin, 115*, 74–101.

Crick, N. R., & Dodge, K. A. (1996). Social information processing mechanisms in reactive and proactive aggression. *Child Development, 67*, 993–1002.

This case study accompanies the textbook: Weis, R. (2021). *Introduction to abnormal child and adolescent psychology* (4th ed.). Thousand Oaks, CA: Sage. Answers appear in the online instructor resources. Visit **https://sagepub.com**.

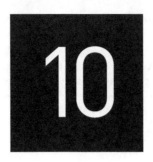

SUBSTANCE USE PROBLEMS IN ADOLESCENTS

CASE STUDY

PATHWAYS TO SUBSTANCE USE PROBLEMS

Preston Allen was referred to the Montgomery County rehabilitation center because of chronic problems with heroin use. Although Preston was only 17 years old, he had a long-standing history of psychosocial stress, disruptive behavior, and substance use problems.

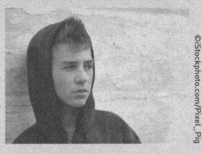

Preston's mother, Gina Herriot, worked as a medical assistant in a local clinic. Preston's father, Mark Allen, held various semiskilled jobs during Preston's childhood and is currently employed in a food processing plant. The couple divorced when Preston was 15 years old, following a tumultuous relationship characterized by frequent verbal arguments and (on two occasions) physical altercations requiring police involvement. Preston's father has a history of arrests ranging from physical assault, breaking and entering, driving while intoxicated, and possession of marijuana with intent to distribute. Preston has little contact with his father today.

As a preschooler, Preston added to his parents' troublesome family life by showing hyperactivity, impulsivity, and inattention. His mother described him as a "risk-taker" and "daredevil" who "couldn't sit still or take no for an answer."

Preston always seemed to be in motion, up to mischief, or doing things to gain the attention of others (either good or bad). A psychological evaluation conducted when Preston was 7 years old also indicated significant oppositional and defiant behavior toward his mother, who reported feeling "totally stressed out" by his hyperactive and noncompliant behavior.

Preston's behavior problems continued into elementary school. He was frequently reprimanded by teachers for talking, leaving his seat, and breaking class rules. He would deliberately annoy classmates, largely to escape the monotony and boredom of the classroom. His classmates came to fear and despise him. Preston was referred to a special education program for children with learning delays and "emotional disturbance." The school counselor's report described him as "a boy whose behavior problems mask underlying feelings of sadness and loneliness." The counselor suggested that his mother become more involved in Preston's schooling, but her hectic work schedule and marital stress interfered with her ability to devote more time to her son.

In junior high school, Preston had been rejected by most youths his age and began associating with older adolescents from the adjacent high school. These new friends, who had behavior problems themselves, introduced Preston to more serious, antisocial acts. Preston began skipping classes, staying out late without his mother's permission, and using nicotine and alcohol. Preston noticed that vaping increased his concentration while, at the same time, reduced tension and anxiety. He used alcohol (and later marijuana) to get "messed up" and enjoy himself with his friends. For the first time in his life, Preston felt like he had a group of friends who liked him "for who he was." Unfortunately, Preston spent considerable time and effort trying to access these substances. As his substance use increased, his school attendance and performance plummeted.

In high school, Preston had begun stealing prescription pain medications from his father and paternal grandmother. He initially used these medications recreationally with his friends. However, he soon began taking them daily to alleviate anxiety and avoid withdrawal symptoms (e.g., headache, nausea, tension). When his father moved out, Preston lost access to these medications. He began using heroin, which he obtained from the "friends of friends" in his neighborhood. Preston became dependent on heroin relatively quickly and used nearly any means necessary to obtain it. At the age of 16, Preston and two young men were arrested for stealing items from parked cars with the intention to sell these items to purchase drugs. Preston was also found in possession of marijuana and prescription medication, which he often sold to high school students to help support his own drug use.

Now 17, Preston was referred for inpatient treatment to help him discontinue heroin and other substances in a controlled, medical environment. "I really want to change," he told the substance abuse counselor who conducted his initial interview. "I'm ready to turn over a new leaf. I hope that you'll give me one more chance to turn my life around."

The counselor reviewed Preston's psychological and medical records. He noticed that Preston had used these same words to describe his situation many times before.

(Continued)

(Continued)

Discussion Questions

1. Review the DSM-5 diagnostic criteria for substance use disorders. Which signs and symptoms does Preston show?

2. How does Preston's psychosocial history reflect the conduct problems pathway for substance use disorders?

3. How does Preston's psychosocial history reflect the negative reinforcement pathway for substance use disorders?

4. How does Preston's psychosocial history reflect the positive reinforcement pathway for substance use disorders?

5. What evidence-based psychosocial treatment might be helpful to adolescents like Preston who have serious substance use problems caused by multiple factors?

This case study accompanies the textbook: Weis, R. (2021). *Introduction to abnormal child and adolescent psychology* (4th ed.). Thousand Oaks, CA: Sage. Answers appear in the online instructor resources. Visit **https://sagepub.com**.

CASE STUDY
MOTIVATIONAL ENHANCEMENT

Irene was a 15-year-old girl referred to mandatory substance abuse counseling by the juvenile court after being arrested for marijuana possession. Approximately 1 month ago, Irene and her friends were caught drinking after a football game in a field a few miles away from her school. Although Irene was not intoxicated, she was questioned by police who discovered a small amount of cannabis in her purse. Whereas her friends were sent home to their parents, Irene was detained by police and ordered by a juvenile court judge to participate in 8 weeks of therapy.

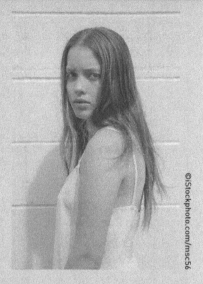

©iStockphoto.com/msc56

"This is total crap," Irene said as she began her first therapy session with Rebecca, her substance use counselor. "Everyone else got to go home, but they arrested me, probably because I was the only Latina. Everyone drinks and uses a little, you know, just to have some fun. God knows we don't go to the games to watch football!"

Rebecca began, cautiously, "Sometimes, adults overreact or do things that are not fair."

Irene replied, "Yeah. There were seven of us and a few boys. All of us drove out there to party and relax. I was the only one who got in trouble."

Rebecca commented, "They singled you out."

"Right. Just me." Irene continued, "And now I'm stuck going to this place. I can think of a dozen kids who drink a lot more than me. Kids who are addicted. Kids who I know sell drugs. But they don't get into trouble. Well if I have to be here, fine. But the judge can't make me talk." Irene crossed her arms in defiance.

Rebecca took a deep breath. She looked away from Irene, out the window, and said, "Your dad tells me you're a good swimmer."

"What?" Irene asked.

Rebecca said, "When I talked to your dad on the telephone before you came here, he mentioned that you swim on the varsity team. He said that you're pretty good and that he's really proud of you."

Puzzled, Irene looked up and replied, "What's that got to do with anything?"

Rebecca explained, "I was wondering... Are you still eligible to swim if you get in trouble with the police?"

(Continued)

[Continued]

Irene replied with a sarcastic tone, "The school swim season doesn't start for 2 months."

"Oh, right," Rebecca said. "But if you get in trouble again, you probably couldn't swim."

Irene paused, digesting Rebecca's words, then responded, "No, probably not."

Rebecca added, "I wonder how your dad would feel if you couldn't swim."

"He'd probably be more hurt by it than I would," Irene replied. "He comes to every meet. He was a college swimmer and really wants me to swim in college too."

Rebecca added, "And you probably like swimming yourself, at least a little? And being on the team?"

Irene answered, "Of course."

Rebecca said, "So even if the police, or the school administrators, or the judge is unfair, or overreacting, or singling you out for whatever reason, it's still in your best interests to NOT get into trouble with alcohol or drugs—at least until swim season is over."

Irene replied, "I guess not."

Discussion Questions

1. What are the six steps in the stages of change model? Which step best describes Irene at the beginning of the session?

2. What are the four overlapping processes of motivational interviewing? Which process did Rebecca emphasize with Irene?

3. What is harm reduction? In what way did Rebecca use a harm reduction approach with Irene?

4. Imagine that you were Irene's therapist. You want to use decision balance to weigh the costs and benefits of (1) continuing her current alcohol and marijuana use versus (2) reducing her substance use. What might be the costs and benefits of each behavior?

5. Irene asserted that most kids her age use alcohol and marijuana regularly. Based on data from the Monitoring the Future studies, is Irene's assertion true? How might Rebecca use individualized feedback to increase Irene's motivation to change?

6. What is the prevalence of substance use problems among Latino adolescents compared to non-Latino White and African American adolescents?

This case study accompanies the textbook: Weis, R. (2021). *Introduction to abnormal child and adolescent psychology* (4th ed.). Thousand Oaks, CA: Sage. Answers appear in the online instructor resources. Visit **https://sagepub.com**.

11

ANXIETY DISORDERS AND OBSESSIVE–COMPULSIVE DISORDER

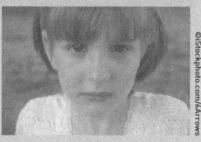

(Continued)

Last year, Liesel began attending preschool approximately three mornings each week while her mother worked part-time. Initially, Liesel was reticent to separate from her mother. However, by the third week of school, she attended preschool without complaining and began to make friends with other girls in her class.

Liesel's school refusal returned at the beginning of this school year, however. The night before the first day of kindergarten, Liesel complained of nausea and stomach pain. When her illness did not subside by the next morning, her mother allowed her to stay home. The following day, when her mother insisted that she attend school, Liesel tantrummed and locked herself in the bathroom. Her mother drove her to school despite protests and crying. Liesel's teacher said that she continued to cry most of the morning and remained tearful and reclusive the rest of the day. When her mother picked her up in the afternoon, Liesel looked hurt and exhausted. She clung to her mother and vowed never to return to school again.

Nevertheless, Liesel's mother insisted that Liesel attend school. Liesel often reported stomach problems, headaches, and other vague illnesses. At school, she behaved in a withdrawn, listless fashion, rarely participating in activities. Liesel also reported transient fears that something bad might happen to her mother or father while she was at school, that terrorists would attack her school, or that her mother might forget to pick her up and that she would have to spend the night alone in the school building.

Liesel's mother reported a significant increase in family stress within the past 6 months, about the time Liesel's school refusal and mood problems emerged. She and her husband are divorcing, which causes her considerable stress and financial hardship. She is struggling to care for her children while also building her interior design business to make ends meet. Liesel's mother admitted to long-standing problems with anxiety and insomnia that have increased markedly since separation from her husband. A second stressor in Liesel's life has been the death of her cat, Tobbie, who was hit by a car outside the family home. Liesel was very attached to Tobbie; she would often hug and pet Tobbie when she was upset. Her mother is considering adopting another cat to replace Tobbie but wondered whether she would have sufficient time and money to care for it.

Discussion Questions

1. What DSM-5 anxiety (or related) disorder best describes Liesel's behavior?

2. Review the DSM-5 criteria for this disorder. Describe how Liesel meets diagnostic criteria for this condition.

3. Liesel is 6 years old. At what age is her problem developmentally normative? Can adolescents experience problems similar to Liesel's?

4. The diathesis stress model is often used to explain the emergence of anxiety disorders. How might the diathesis stress model be used to explain the development of Liesel's problems with school refusal?

5. What evidence-based treatment might you recommend for Liesel?

This case study accompanies the textbook: Weis, R. (2021). *Introduction to abnormal child and adolescent psychology* (4th ed.). Thousand Oaks, CA: Sage. Answers appear in the online instructor resources. Visit **https://sagepub.com**.

CASE STUDY
TACITURN TESS

Mrs. Miller sat awkwardly in the small desk of her daughter's kindergarten classroom. As she shifted her weight, she waited for her daughter's teacher, Ms. Shafer, to speak.

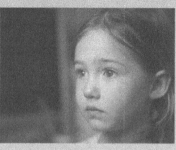

"Thank you for meeting with me today," said Ms. Shafer. "I'm glad that we can talk about your daughter, Tessa."

"Of course," Mrs. Miller responded. "Is there a problem?"

The teacher replied, "Tessa's a delight to have in class. She's always attentive and completes her work in a neat, organized way. Her spelling and math are coming along nicely, too. There's just one concern—she doesn't talk much."

This report was not what Mrs. Miller was expecting. Confused, she asked, "What do you mean? She talks all the time at home."

Ms. Shafer answered, "We've been in school for 6 weeks. Tessa's never said a word. She's definitely gotten better since the first day of school. In August, she wouldn't even make eye contact with me. She'd just sit at her desk or stand on the fringes of group activities and refuse to participate. Now, she'll look me in the eye when I talk to her and answer questions by nodding or shaking her head. I still can't assess her reading skills because she refuses to read aloud in class or in her reading circle." Ms. Shafer paused and then asked, "Is anything wrong at home? Is she under a lot of stress or did something bad happen?"

Mrs. Miller was stunned. She responded, "No. Nothing's really changed at our house." She thought to herself for a while and added, "Tessa's always been a very shy girl. My husband called her 'shadow' because she's constantly by our side. She even dislikes being in the living room alone and insists that one of us is with her. She's also had a hard time making friends, but has a few younger kids in the neighborhood that she likes."

Ms. Shafer questioned, "What was Tessa like last year in school?"

"Actually," Mrs. Miller began, "Tessa didn't attend formal school because our family was traveling due to my husband's work. He's a petroleum engineer and our family spent last year in South America. I homeschooled Tessa because other schooling options were limited. Maybe that was a mistake."

Ms. Shafer replied, "Like I said, Tessa is making progress—although it's not as fast as I would like. I think we can help her overcome this problem, but we need to work together."

Discussion Questions

1. What DSM-5 anxiety (or related) disorder best describes Tessa's behavior?

2. Review the DSM-5 criteria for this disorder. Describe how Tessa meets diagnostic criteria for this condition.

(Continued)

(Continued)

3. Tessa is a kindergarten student. At what age do problems like hers typically emerge? If untreated, is she likely to get better by herself?

4. How might temperament play a role in Tessa's difficulty at school?

5. How might we use learning theory to explain the cause and maintenance of Tessa's problem?

6. What evidence-based treatment might you recommend for Tessa?

This case study accompanies the textbook: Weis, R. (2021). *Introduction to abnormal child and adolescent psychology* (4th ed.). Thousand Oaks, CA: Sage. Answers appear in the online instructor resources. Visit **https://sagepub.com**.

CASE STUDY
DENTAL PLAN

Nora was a 10-year-old girl who was referred to our outpatient clinic because of persistent fears about going to the dentist. Nora's problems began approximately 6 months ago following a routine dental procedure that ended up in disaster.

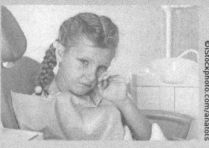

©iStockphoto.com/anatols

Nora was a typically developing fourth-grader who was well behaved at home, a good student, and popular with classmates. She had no history of anxiety or mood disorders in her family and was physically healthy. Consequently, when Nora's mother took her to the dentist to fill a small cavity, she did not expect the visit to go so poorly.

As the dentist began drilling to remove portions of the decayed tooth, Nora felt the dull pressure of the machine against her jaw and inhaled the burnt aroma of bone against the drill tip. As the scent assailed her nostrils, she experienced saliva filling the lower portion of her mouth, sliding rapidly toward her throat. She thought, "I need to swallow. I'm going to drown in my own spit. I need to get it out, but I can't." Nora was too embarrassed to ask the dentist to pause and allow her to swallow. She felt her eyes tear, her face and neck broke out in a cold sweat, and her heart began to thump. Then, she began to choke. The drill slipped and injured her tooth, saliva flew in all directions, and Nora vomited a little on her clothes. An overwhelming sense of embarrassment flooded Nora. She felt a terrible impulse to run from the exam room and, without thinking, she bolted. Her mother watched her run down the hallway, past her seat in the waiting room, and out the door. After 20 minutes of heavy sobbing, Nora explained what happened.

Nora has since refused to visit the dentist. Her mother has tried to take her to different offices, but Nora either cries, tantrums, or stubbornly refuses to enter. Her mother is concerned because Nora's cavity was never filled and she is still in need of dental work. Her mother is hoping that a psychologist might develop a plan to help Nora muster the courage to visit the dentist.

Discussion Questions

1. What DSM-5 anxiety (or related) disorder best describes Nora's behavior?

2. Review the DSM-5 criteria for this disorder. Describe how Nora meets diagnostic criteria for this condition.

3. How do older children and adolescents' fears differ from the fears of preschool- and young school-age children?

(Continued)

(Continued)

4. How might Nora's cognitions mediate the relationship between her situation (i.e., the dental procedure) and her emotional and behavioral consequences (e.g., fear/panic and fleeing the office)?

5. How might we use learning theory to explain the cause and maintenance of Nora's problem?

6. What evidence-based treatment might you recommend for Nora?

This case study accompanies the textbook: Weis, R. (2021). *Introduction to abnormal child and adolescent psychology* (4th ed.). Thousand Oaks, CA: Sage. Answers appear in the online instructor resources. Visit **https://sagepub.com**.

CASE STUDY
GUN-SHY GUY

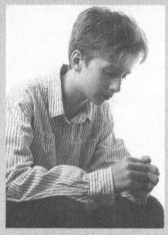

Logan Wright was a handsome, intelligent, tenth-grade student at Watkins High School. Although Logan was somewhat quiet and reserved, he had a small circle of close friends and was involved in the school's marching band. Logan was also an excellent student, earning mostly As in advanced courses in math and science. Overall, Logan was successfully navigating the world of adolescence, except for one small problem: he could not urinate in a public restroom.

Logan's problem was discovered by his teacher several days ago when he left his classroom during a test without permission. Apparently, Logan had refrained from using the bathroom all day and drank too much fluid to delay urination any longer. After 20 minutes of uncomfortable fidgeting, Logan darted from the classroom down the hall to the bathroom. Although no one stood at the urinals, one student occupied a nearby stall. Logan quickly exited the bathroom and dashed to a different bathroom at the other end of the school. Luckily, no one was inside the second bathroom and Logan could relieve his bladder. However, he had some explaining to do.

"How long have you had this problem?" his school counselor asked.

"Forever," Logan replied. "At first, it wasn't much of a problem. I would always just pee in a stall. Then, about 3 years ago, it became worse and I couldn't pee if anyone was in the bathroom."

The counselor asked, "What is it about peeing in public that bothers you?"

Logan laughed nervously and then replied, "I don't know. I guess I'm worried that someone will hear me. I know it's really dumb, but I think that they might be making fun of me."

"What might they think?" the counselor asked.

"I don't know. Maybe that I pee really loud or that I pee different from others or maybe that they'll be looking at me funny. I know it's silly, but when I have these thoughts I tense up and can't go."

The counselor asked, "Have you ever told anyone about this problem, like your dad?"

Logan laughed cynically and then said, "No. He's not the type of person to go to with a problem like this."

"What do you mean?" asked the counselor.

(Continued)

(Continued)

"I mean, he's not the most understanding person in the world," Logan explained. "Let's just say we don't have a good relationship."

"And I don't suppose you can talk to your mom about a problem like this," said the counselor.

Logan replied, "Not really. Besides, she's a bundle of nerves herself. She's been taking anxiety medication for years."

The counselor responded, "Well, I'm glad that we can talk about it. Let's see if we can find a way to help you get over this problem."

Discussion Questions

1. What DSM-5 anxiety (or related) disorder best describes Logan's behavior?

2. Review the DSM-5 criteria for this disorder. Describe how Logan meets diagnostic criteria for this condition.

3. Logan is a tenth-grade student (perhaps 15 years of age). At what age do youths with his disorder typically manifest symptoms?

4. Logan seems to have a negative attitude toward his father and his mother. According to the research literature, how can parents contribute to the development of anxiety disorders in children?

5. How might a behavior therapist use graded exposure to help Logan overcome his problem?

6. What cognitive distortions might contribute to Logan's anxiety problem? How might a cognitive therapist address these distortions?

This case study accompanies the textbook: Weis, R. (2021). *Introduction to abnormal child and adolescent psychology* (4th ed.). Thousand Oaks, CA: Sage. Answers appear in the online instructor resources. Visit **https://sagepub.com**.

CASE STUDY
CARDIO CONSULT

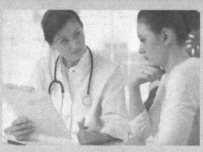

©iStockphoto.com/AlexRaths

Sivan sat in the cardiologist's office with her parents. Her mother sat by her side with her arm around the back of Sivan's chair. Her father sat nervously across from them, periodically rubbing his forehead. Sivan was their only child. Sixteen years ago, she was born with a congenital heart defect that threatened her life and necessitated a series of operations that kept her in and out of hospitals for most of her infancy. Her parents thought that all of these medical problems were in Sivan's past. Sivan had not experienced any irregularities in years and had even been cleared to play tennis and ride horses (activities that she adored). Then, several months ago, all of that changed.

Sivan was completing an important chemistry exam when she experienced severe heart palpitations. The palpitations came on suddenly, as if her heart skipped a beat. They were accompanied with a curious "sinking feeling" like she was going to faint. She later described it as similar to the time when she was pulled over by the police for speeding. She felt dizzy and lightheaded, experienced shortness of breath, and her skin felt clammy. Immediately, Sivan left the classroom without permission, ran to an empty adjacent room, and curled into a ball on the floor waiting to feel better. After about 20 minutes, she was able to walk to the bathroom and wash her face. She returned to her classroom, explained to her teacher that she felt sick, and put the event behind her.

Unfortunately, Sivan experienced similar episodes over the subsequent 3 months. Three episodes occurred at school, usually before or during exams. One episode, however, happened in the school parking lot as she was walking to her car to drive home. This last episode greatly upset Sivan because it came "out of the blue," it did not seem prompted by stress, and it could have been dangerous if it had occurred while she was driving. Worried about their recurrence, Sivan told her parents about these events and they immediately contacted her pediatrician who ordered testing.

"I have the results of Sivan's EEG," said the cardiologist. "The good news is that it looks completely normal. I don't think she's experiencing any return of the problems she's had in the past."

Her father let out a sigh of relief, followed by the inevitable question, "But then why is Sivan having these episodes?"

"And how can we stop them?" added her mother.

(Continued)

[Continued]

Discussion Questions

1. What DSM-5 anxiety (or related) disorder best describes Sivan's behavior?

2. Review the DSM-5 criteria for this disorder. Describe how Sivan meets diagnostic criteria for this condition.

3. How might expectancy theory be used to explain the development of Sivan's symptoms?

4. According to a cognitive therapist, how might Sivan's thoughts contribute to her recurrent problem?

5. What evidence-based interventions might a therapist use to help Sivan?

This case study accompanies the textbook: Weis, R. (2021). *Introduction to abnormal child and adolescent psychology* (4th ed.). Thousand Oaks, CA: Sage. Answers appear in the online instructor resources. Visit **https://sagepub.com**.

CASE STUDY
STOMACH PROBLEMS

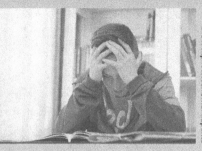

©iStockphoto.com/martiapunts

Luke Atkins was a 13-year-old boy referred to our outpatient clinic because of problems with social avoidance. Luke's mother, Margaret Atkins, works as a defense attorney. His father, Bill Atkins, works as an accountant. Luke has two younger sisters and no family history of mental health problems. Prior to the onset of his current anxiety problem, Luke had been a friendly, although somewhat introverted boy, who did well in school, liked to play soccer, and had a close group of friends.

Six months ago, Luke's mother received a telephone call from the school nurse who reported that Luke was involved in an "incident" at school. After lunch, Luke experienced upset stomach, cramping, and heartburn. He attempted to cope with these symptoms by sitting quietly at his desk. When the discomfort increased, Luke asked his teacher if he could be excused because he was not feeling well. As Luke rose from his desk, Luke felt a surge of stomach acid and partially undigested food enter the back of his mouth. He gagged and, embarrassingly, regurgitated some of the contents onto his shirt and the floor. Luke ran from the room to the nurse's office.

The following day, Luke refused to go to school, claiming that he was too embarrassed to show his face to his classmates. Only after much coaxing were his parents able to persuade him to go. Unfortunately, later that week, Luke experienced another attack of upset stomach that almost caused him to vomit in the same classroom. This time, however, Luke left the classroom in time and took antacids, which alleviated his symptoms.

Luke's pediatrician prescribed medication for acid reflux and recommended that he carry antacids with him during the day at school. Nevertheless, Luke refused to attend his afternoon math class, so school personnel rearranged his schedule. Luke experienced minor acid reflux problems over the next few weeks: at first period physical education class, immediately after lunch in his new language arts class, and on the bus ride home. This last incident was especially problematic. Luke, who was formerly so self-reliant, insisted that his mother pick him up from school in case he experienced another stomach problem on the bus and could not get to the bathroom or otherwise obtain help.

Currently, Luke complains about going to school each morning. He refuses to eat lunch at school because he is afraid of more attacks. School personnel have rearranged his schedule a third time so that his "important" classes (e.g., math, language arts) are in the morning when he is likely to feel well. Luke attends his afternoon classes very reluctantly and insists that he sit near the door in case he

(Continued)

(Continued)

needs to leave in an emergency. He refuses to attend physical education class. His parents have rearranged their work schedules so they can drive him home each afternoon.

Luke denies other symptoms of anxiety or mood problems. He says that he has never experienced a panic attack and is not afraid of social situations. His chief worry is that his stomach problems will become worse, thus limiting his functioning even more.

Discussion Questions

1. What DSM-5 anxiety (or related) disorder best describes Luke's behavior?

2. Review the DSM-5 criteria for this disorder. Describe how Luke meets diagnostic criteria for this condition.

3. How common are problems like the kind experienced by Luke (e.g., avoiding school, the bus)? At what age do problems like Luke's tend to emerge?

4. Approximately what percentage of youths have problems like Luke without a history of panic attacks?

5. According to Mowrer's two-factor theory of anxiety, how did Luke's avoidance of class and the bus emerge? Why has it persisted over time?

6. Imagine that you are a cognitive therapist. How might you help Luke?

This case study accompanies the textbook: Weis, R. (2021). *Introduction to abnormal child and adolescent psychology* (4th ed.). Thousand Oaks, CA: Sage. Answers appear in the online instructor resources. Visit **https://sagepub.com**.

CASE STUDY
TALENTED MUSICIAN

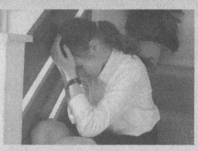

Chloe McGovern was referred to the pediatric headache clinic at a children's hospital in a metropolitan area. Chloe was a 13-year-old, eighth-grade student with tension headaches of moderate intensity. The headaches began approximately 18 months ago and have gradually worsened, especially over the past 6 months. These headaches occurred approximately 3 times per week, with a duration of approximately 1 to 3 hours each. Over-the-counter medications (e.g., acetaminophen, ibuprofen) are generally effective in shortening their duration but Chloe's parents are worried, given the increasing frequency and severity of the headaches.

A neurological examination revealed no abnormalities that might explain the headaches. Consequently, Chloe and her family were referred to a pediatric psychologist at the clinic to explore psychosocial causes for her problem. The psychologist, Dr. Witten, learned that the onset of Chloe's headaches coincided with her transition to middle school.

Chloe's mother explained, "Chloe's always been a perfectionist. She was in accelerated programs throughout elementary school: math, language arts, music. When she started middle school, she tested into the gifted program, meaning that she could skip seventh-grade classes and begin eighth-grade work for most subjects."

Her father added, "And she's also a very good musician. They asked her to play for both the seventh- and eighth-grade orchestras. She plays the oboe, which is somewhat rare. Both orchestras needed her."

Dr. Witten looked up from her notes, "And is all this work hard to manage, Chloe? I mean, you skipped seventh grade."

Chloe answered, "Not really." Then crossed her arms and remained silent.

Chloe's mother elaborated, "Chloe's a hard worker. I drive her to school each morning a little early because she's on the student council. She tries to do as much homework as possible during study hall. Then, after school, she has orchestra or archery practice. She also takes private oboe lessons twice a week."

"That's a busy schedule," commented Dr. Witten. Chloe remained silent. Later, Dr. Witten interviewed Chloe privately.

She said, "Chloe, I know that you're a good musician. I wonder if you're a good artist, too. I want you to draw me a picture of yourself just when your headache is about to begin. Draw how you feel." Reluctantly, Chloe sketched the image of a teenage girl with taut shoulders, a stiff neck, a bulging forehead and eyes, and a worried expression on her face.

(Continued)

(Continued)

Dr. Witten responded, "That's an interesting picture. The girl looks so tense! I wonder what's going through her mind." Dr. Witten drew a bubble above the image of the girl and then asked, "Write some words that describe what she's thinking."

Chloe hesitated, reached for the pencil, paused again, and then began writing. The words flowed from her, like water breaking through an old dam that was no longer able to bear the strain: *math test, language arts presentation, student council service project, science fair, wind ensemble, dad's cholesterol, mom's work schedule, friends, another headache, getting enough sleep, grandma's sick. . . .*

"Do you think about these things before you have a headache?" asked Dr. Witten.

Chloe looked up from the paper, then answered, "I think about these things all of the time. There's always something going on in my life, something to worry about. I tell myself, 'Relax. Nobody else worries about things like you do.' But it doesn't do any good. I feel tense all the time. I can't control it. It's the worst at night, before I fall asleep. All of the things I need to do or should have done come to my mind and they don't stop."

Dr. Witten responded, "All the things that you're good at, like school and music?"

"Right," Chloe sighed. As a tear trickled down her cheek, she added, "That's just it. I think that if I didn't worry so much—you know, make sure I've planned for everything—I might not get good grades, or do well in my ensembles, or make mom and dad happy."

Dr. Witten pointed to her head and replied, "You carry all this pressure up here. Your problem is not the headaches, though—it's that you think too much! I'd like to work with you to find a way to stop all that worrying. Would you like that?"

For the first time in a long time, Chloe smiled.

Discussion Questions

1. What DSM-5 anxiety (or associated) disorder best describes Chloe's behavior?

2. How does Chloe meet DSM-5 criteria for this disorder?

3. When do problems with worrying tend to emerge? Is Chloe's age of onset developmentally typical?

4. Chloe seems to worry about mundane things: school, extracurricular activities, family. How does the worrying of children with anxiety disorders differ from the worrying of typically developing children?

5. Chloe seems to be a high-achieving girl who is rather mature for her age. Is this typical of children with anxiety disorders?

6. Based on the results of longitudinal studies, what disorder is Chloe at particular risk for developing as she enters later adolescence and early adulthood?

7. How can cognitive-avoidance theory be used to explain Chloe's problem with chronic worrying?

8. If you were Chloe's clinician, what evidence-based psychotherapies or pharmacological interventions might you recommend?

This case study accompanies the textbook: Weis, R. (2021). *Introduction to abnormal child and adolescent psychology* (4th ed.). Thousand Oaks, CA: Sage. Answers appear in the online instructor resources. Visit **https://sagepub.com**.

CASE STUDY
SIBLING RIVALRY

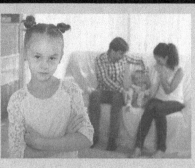

©iStockphoto.com/JackF

Isabella Hague was an 11-year-old girl referred to an outpatient mental health clinic by her mother because of "a curious preoccupation about harming her infant brother." Isabella's immediate family consisted of herself, her father and mother, and her 12-month-old baby brother, Manuel. Isabella's mother, a sales executive, and her father, a store manager, were thrilled when Isabella was born. The couple had difficulty conceiving a child. Although they thought Isabella would be their only child, Mrs. Hague was surprised to learn that she was pregnant with Manuel last year. Mrs. Hague reduced her work hours to stay at home with Manuel and the family soon adjusted to being a group of four.

Or so it seemed. Approximately 3 months after Manuel's birth, Mrs. Hague noticed Isabella's mood change. The formerly cheerful girl who loved to spend time with her parents became irritable and reclusive.

"Isabella would often snap at us for no reason," described her mother. "She'd seldom smile and was often crabby or disrespectful. We knew something was different about her. She'd also spend a lot of time by herself, usually in her room or in her tree house in the backyard."

Mr. Hague added, "We figured that Isabella was having a bad case of sibling rivalry. For 11 years, she was our only child—our baby. Now she has to share attention with Manny. And, to be honest, Manny demands a lot of attention. We tried to make sure that Isabella didn't feel neglected, so we'd take her on special outings, like to the movies or to dinner—you know, one-on-one."

On one such outing, Mrs. Hague discovered the source of Isabella's change in mood. While they were eating frozen custard, Mrs. Hague raised the possibility that Isabella might be jealous of Manny. Isabella burst into tears. After a long while, Isabella admitted that she often had "strange thoughts" about hurting Manny. Once, while watching Manny in his crib, Isabella thought about how easy it would be to smother him with a blanket or pillow. Another time, when her mother was bathing Manny, Isabella imagined drowning him in the tub. Such thoughts began shortly after his birth and gradually increased in frequency and severity.

The psychologist at the clinic questioned Isabella about her strange thoughts. Isabella explained, "I love Manny so much. I've always wanted a baby brother or sister. I'd never do anything to hurt him. I feel so guilty!"

"Guilty?" the psychologist asked.

"Like maybe I might actually do something that could hurt him," Isabella explained. "I know I never will but I still think about it." She paused and then added, "Like maybe if I think about it, it might actually come true."

(Continued)

(Continued)

The psychologist asked, "So if you don't act upon these thoughts, how do you get rid of them?"

Isabella responded hesitantly, "I pray. I ask God to get rid of these bad thoughts and to help me love my brother. I know I shouldn't have these thoughts, but I do, so I pray to get rid of them."

"Do you say specific prayers?" asked the psychologist.

"At first I would say three Our Fathers," said Isabella. "That helped a lot. Then I started adding other prayers to get the thoughts out of my mind and to make me feel better. This all took a lot of time and if I messed up, I'd think, 'I need to start over and get it right' otherwise it wouldn't work."

"You mean, if you didn't say the prayers right, it wouldn't help you get rid of the bad thoughts?" asked the psychologist.

"Yes," responded Isabella. "Or it wouldn't stop bad things from happening to Manny. Sometimes, I would spend a lot of time praying, getting it right until I felt like everything was okay. I wish there was some way I could stop."

Discussion Questions

1. What DSM-5 anxiety (or related) disorder best describes Isabella's behavior?

2. Review the DSM-5 criteria for this disorder. Describe how Isabella meets diagnostic criteria for this condition.

3. How might you characterize Isabella's *insight* regarding her problem?

4. What two cognitive distortions often characterize the thoughts of children and adolescents with Isabella's condition? Does Isabella experience these cognitive distortions?

5. What is PANDAS? Is it applicable to Isabella?

This case study accompanies the textbook: Weis, R. (2021). *Introduction to abnormal child and adolescent psychology* (4th ed.). Thousand Oaks, CA: Sage. Answers appear in the online instructor resources. Visit **https://sagepub.com**.

CASE STUDY
CAN'T FIGHT THIS FEELING

David Simons was an 8-year-old boy referred to an outpatient mental health clinic by his pediatrician because of chronic anxiety and "nervous habits." David is the only child of Joseph and Margaret Simons. Mr. Simons works as a house painter. Mrs. Simons recently returned to work as a medical technician after several years of caring for David at home.

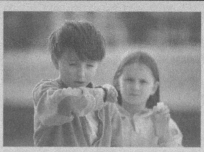

Approximately 18 months ago, David's parents brought him to his pediatrician because of an upper respiratory infection. Although David recovered from this illness, his parents noticed lingering problems with sniffling, wrinkling and wiping his nose, and a persistent, dry cough. A follow-up appointment showed David to be healthy. His physician suggested that David might have developed some "bad habits" during his illness that would likely go away over time.

David's strange mannerisms subsided over the following weeks, only to return with greater intensity at the beginning of the school year. During his first weeks of kindergarten, David began coughing again, approximately 30 times per hour. His coughs were accompanied with head turns, rapid blinking, and a grimace that resembled a combination of a smirk and a wink. These mannerisms gradually waned over the first 3 months of school.

David's cough and repetitive facial movements returned yet a third time several months ago. This time, their onset coincided with his mother's return to full-time employment and David's enrollment in an after-school program. David's classmates began to tease him, calling him names like "coughy" and "sicky" and running away from him as if he had a contagious disease. David's teacher allowed David to leave the classroom when he felt the need to cough. This strategy reduced class disruptions but caused David to miss out on learning.

The psychologist who conducted the evaluation learned that Mr. Simons had a history of obsessive–compulsive behavior in early adolescence. His condition was never diagnosed and gradually improved on its own. Mrs. Simons denied obsessions or compulsions, but she admitted to chronic problems with anxiety and insomnia for which she takes medication.

David said, "I just can't help myself" when he coughs, turns his head, wrinkles his nose, blinks, or winks. Just before he coughs, he gets a "strange feeling, like something building up inside" that he "just has to let go." David says that if he tries to fight the urge, it gets worse until he "can't hold it back." David denied having any thoughts, ideas, or images before coughing. He admitted that he felt "bad" about disrupting class and reported that he felt sad and lonely at school. Neither

(Continued)

(Continued)

David's parents nor his teacher reported problems with hyperactivity or inattention. However, his parents and teacher noticed increased problems with sadness and social withdrawal.

Discussion Questions

1. What DSM-5 anxiety (or related) disorder best describes David's behavior?

2. Explain how David meets DSM-5 diagnostic criteria for this condition.

3. How might a clinician differentiate David's condition from OCD?

4. Does David still meet diagnostic criteria for this disorder, despite the absence of coprolalia?

5. Is it typical for children to show a waxing and waning of symptoms over time, as displayed by David? What causes this waxing and waning?

6. In the case study, the psychologist assessed David for OCD. Is it possible for David to also have OCD?

7. If you were David's psychologist, what evidence-based treatments might you recommend?

This case study accompanies the textbook: Weis, R. (2021). *Introduction to abnormal child and adolescent psychology* (4th ed.). Thousand Oaks, CA: Sage. Answers appear in the online instructor resources. Visit **https://sagepub.com**.

12

TRAUMA-RELATED DISORDERS

CASE STUDY
HURT INSIDE

Ivy Minton was a 24-month-old toddler referred to our clinic by her foster mother, Jennifer Spencer. Ms. Spencer is a foster parent who had been caring for Ivy for the past 3 months alongside her three other foster children. Ivy was removed from her parents' custody several months earlier due to child endangerment and neglect. Ivy 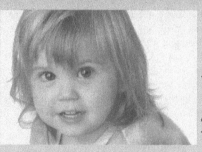 was discovered, unsupervised, in a dilapidated apartment. Her mother had a history of opioid dependence. The paramedics were called to the apartment by Ivy's aunt who reported that Ivy's mother had overdosed on heroin.

Child Protective Services sought an emergency foster placement for Ivy with her maternal grandmother. However, chronic health problems interfered with her grandmother's ability to care for Ivy. After 6 weeks in her grandmother's care, Ivy was again relocated, this time to Ms. Spencer's foster home. Although her long-term treatment plan involves parental reunification, Ivy's mother has experienced problems recovering from her substance use problem.

Developmental rating scales, completed by Ms. Spencer, indicated that Ivy's motor, cognitive, and adaptive functioning were within normal limits for a child her age. Physically, Ivy was healthy. Although she exhibited minor problems with

(Continued)

(Continued)

insomnia and occasional picky eating, her foster mother reported no problems with her affect and mood. Her social functioning, however, caused her foster mother concern.

"Two weeks ago was the final straw. Me, Ivy, and two of the other kids were playing in the park. I was helping Ivy down the little slide and she scraped her leg as she came down. She screamed something awful! Then, she walked past me and ran toward another mom, begging to be picked up. The other mom gave me a strange look, bent down, and picked up Ivy to comfort her. I thought, 'Why didn't Ivy come to me? Aren't I the one who's been caring for her all these months? What am I doing wrong?' What surprised me even more is when the other mom tried to return Ivy to me. Ivy fussed, like she didn't want to leave the other mom. My initial feeling of embarrassment was replaced by a deep hurt inside."

Ms. Spencer described similar episodes of Ivy's overly social behavior. During playdates and church activities, Ivy seemed just as content sitting next to other parents as her foster mother. On one occasion, she hopped onto the youth pastor's lap and began stroking his beard in an affectionate way, much to his surprise and embarrassment. Ivy wandered off with adults she did not know on two occasions. "She gave me quite a scare," commented Ms. Spencer. "I need to watch her like a hawk because she'll go off with anyone—even strangers—without checking with me first."

Observations of Ms. Spencer and Ivy in the clinic playroom confirmed her foster mother's reports. Ivy was an active, verbal, 2-year-old who took delight in social engagement. She maintained good eye contact and showed appropriate imitation and imaginary play. She also displayed adequate reciprocity in her social interactions and a high degree of positive affect. Ivy's motor skills were within normal limits. Although she fussed slightly when Ms. Spencer told her it was time to clean up, Ivy responded well to her foster mother's directions. Curiously, Ivy showed no anxiety when she first met the psychologist and readily went off with the receptionist to another room when the psychologist and Ms. Spencer discussed treatment options.

Discussion Questions

1. What DSM-5 disorder best describes Ivy's behavior?

2. How does Ivy meet diagnostic criteria for this condition?

3. How does Ivy exhibit both risk and resilience?

4. What is an underlying cause of Ivy's problems in social functioning?

5. What is Ivy's prognosis, assuming she receives treatment?

6. What evidence-based treatments are effective for youths like Ivy?

This case study accompanies the textbook: Weis, R. (2021). *Introduction to abnormal child and adolescent psychology* (4th ed.). Thousand Oaks, CA: Sage. Answers appear in the online instructor resources. Visit **https://sagepub.com**.

CASE STUDY
WALMART TROUBLES

Most children who experience physical or psychological maltreatment are not permanently removed from their parents' homes. A primary goal of therapy is to help parents manage negative thoughts and feelings so that they can care for their children in more supportive and less hostile ways. Parent–child cognitive–behavioral therapy

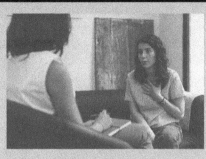
©iStockphoto.com/FilippoBacci

(PC-CBT) is an evidence-based approach to teaching parents these skills and preventing future abuse and neglect (Runyon & Deblinger, 2019).

In this passage, a therapist helps a parent see the connection between her thoughts, feelings, and actions toward her children. As you read the passage, notice how the therapist helps the parent identify and change potentially maladaptive thoughts that might lead to maltreatment.

Therapist: You've shared with me how stressful it can be to parent three daughters. Now, let's look at a situation with your children to see if we can make your job as a parent less stressful. Tell me about a time when you felt angry or frustrated with your children this week.

Parent: We went to Walmart to buy some book bags and they threw a fit because I would not buy the expensive ones they wanted. So I yelled at them and left without any of the bags.

Therapist: On a scale of 1 to 10, how stressed or angry were you?

Parent: When I yelled at the kids, my anger level was a 9.

Therapist: Let's look at the situation more closely. Imagine that you are in the situation right now. What happened right before you became angry?

Parent: Well, I gave them a choice between two cheaper bags, but they didn't want those. They wanted the expensive ones so they whined and complained. They always want everything we can't afford. I don't know why they can't be happy. Anyway, I told them to choose between the two bags or we would leave with none.

Therapist: What were you thinking to yourself when you gave them a choice?

(Continued)

[Continued]

Parent: I was thinking: Here we go again. They always want more than we can afford. They are so ungrateful. I work my butt off to get them what they need, but they don't appreciate it.

Therapist: What happened next?

Parent: They didn't choose. They demanded the expensive bags. So I got mad at them and yelled.

Therapist: What were you thinking to yourself just before you yelled?

Parent: I was thinking that these are the most ungrateful kids in the world. I also thought that they might act that way in public just to embarrass me.

Therapist: What did you do?

Parent: I got mad at them and yelled. I told them they were ungrateful and that they didn't deserve the bags at all. I told them I should drop them off at CPS (Child Protective Services) and let them be someone else's problem.

Therapist: It sounds like you were really angry and stressed out. Let's go back and see what you did well in the situation and what you could have done differently. First, you gave them a clear choice about what bags they *could* have. You also clearly stated what the consequence would be if they did not choose. That was great! I mean that's textbook parenting! Now, let's see if there's anything you could have done differently.

Parent: Well, I really wish I hadn't become angry and yelled at them.

Therapist: Yes. We've already talked about how our thoughts, feelings, and actions are connected. We can change our feelings and actions by changing our thoughts. How could you have thought about the situation differently?

Parent: I could have told myself that I can stay calm and handle this. I also could have told myself that they are just kids and do not understand finances.

Therapist: That's great! Is there anything else you might have done differently?

Parent: I could have told them that they were not going to get the expensive bags and left the store without arguing with them.

Therapist: How would you have felt?

Parent: I wouldn't have become so angry, said mean things, and regretted it later.

Discussion Questions

1. The first phase of PC-CBT is engagement. How did the therapist try to engage the parent in this session?

2. The second phase of PC-CBT is skill building. Most therapists use the antecedent-belief-consequence (ABC) model to show parents that their beliefs about antecedent events, rather than the events themselves, cause them to act and feel in certain ways. Use the following table to complete the ABC model for the parent in the passage.

Antecedent	Belief	Consequence

3. Another technique used by cognitive–behavioral therapists is to help parents identify and challenge cognitive distortions that cause them to feel angry, to lose their temper, or to act in hostile or coercive ways toward their children. What cognitive distortion(s) did the parent report in the session and how might the therapist challenge these beliefs?

4. A final technique used by cognitive–behavioral therapists is to improve parents' emotional coping skills. How might the therapist improve the emotion-regulation skills of the parent in this session?

Reference

Runyon, M. K., & Deblinger, E. (2019). *Combined parent–child cognitive behavioral therapy.* New York, NY: Oxford.

This case study accompanies the textbook: Weis, R. (2021). *Introduction to abnormal child and adolescent psychology* (4th ed.). Thousand Oaks, CA: Sage. Answers appear in the online instructor resources. Visit **https://sagepub.com**.

CASE STUDY

MOCKINGJAY

Katniss Everdeen is a 17-year-old girl from District 12, a coal-mining region that is the poorest and least populated district in the dystopian nation of Panem. Katniss volunteered to replace her sister, Primrose ("Prim"), after she was chosen to compete in the Hunger Games, a televised fight to the death. Katniss and Peeta Mellark (a boy from her district) eventually win the Hunger Games after all the other participants are killed by each other

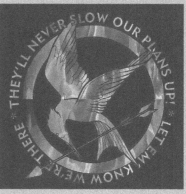

Image courtesy of Presidenvolksraad Wikimedia Commons

or mishaps in the Arena. During the course of the Games, Katniss witnesses other teenagers killing each other with knives, axes, bows, and other weapons. She also witnesses the death of her 12-year-old friend, Rue, at the hands of another contestant.

Since the Hunger Games, Katniss and Peeta have been living in Victors' Village, a more luxurious area of District 12. Katniss and her family are no longer starving. Nevertheless, Katniss is not doing well. She seldom talks about events that occurred during the Games and has cut off all contact with her mentors who helped her prepare for the contest. She also avoids Peeta, despite the fact that he lives only a few houses away. At home, Katniss is often irritable and prone to angry outbursts. She seems constantly on edge and on the lookout, as if she expects bad things to happen. She's easily startled, too. Once, when Prim's cat unexpectedly jumped on her bed, Katniss screamed and instinctively threw a bottle at it!

Katniss suffers from insomnia almost every night and will often sleep with her sister in order to feel safe. On several occasions, Katniss has experienced nightmares: either about events that occurred during the Games or other dreams with macabre, violent themes. When hunting deer with her boyfriend, Gale, Katniss also momentarily believed that she shot another teenager in the Arena rather than the deer. When Gale asked her about this, Katniss refused to discuss it with him and this strained their relationship.

Indeed, Katniss's relationship with Gale has deteriorated significantly since her return from the Hunger Games. Although they used to love each other, Katniss now shows little affection toward him. When Gale asked Katniss if she loves him, Katniss replied, "All I can think about every day since the Games is how afraid I am. There is no room for anything else." Although Katniss does not report feeling depressed, she seems unable to experience joy or pleasure in anything. Even hunting, which she formerly enjoyed, now only brings unwanted memories. Although she would never admit it to anyone else, Katniss often thinks that maybe it should have been her, not Rue, who died in the Games.

On several occasions, Katniss has thought about using alcohol or painkillers to help her cope. However, she has refrained from using substances like these because her family relies on her for their well-being. "Besides," Katniss admits, "I don't want to wind up like Haymitch."

Discussion Question

Does Katniss meet DSM-5 diagnostic criteria for PTSD? Review each of the diagnostic criteria below and determine which she satisfies.

A. Exposure to actual or threatened death, serious injury, or sexual violence.

B. One (or more) intrusion symptoms associated with the traumatic event.

C. Persistent avoidance of stimuli associated with the traumatic event.

D. Negative alterations in cognitions and mood associated with the traumatic event as evidenced by two (or more) signs or symptoms.

E. Marked alterations in arousal and reactivity associated with the traumatic event as evidenced by two (or more) signs or symptoms.

F. The duration of the disturbance is more than 1 month.

G. The disturbance causes clinically significant distress or impairment.

H. The disturbance is not attributable to the physiological effects of a substance or another medical condition.

This case study accompanies the textbook: Weis, R. (2021). *Introduction to abnormal child and adolescent psychology* (4th ed.). Thousand Oaks, CA: Sage. Answers appear in the online instructor resources. Visit **https://sagepub.com**.

CASE STUDY
FAMILY PROBLEMS

Henry Evans was an 11-year-old boy referred to outpatient therapy by Child Protective Services. Henry is the oldest of four children born to Mark Evans and Julia Bryers. His younger sisters (aged 6 and 9 years, respectively) and brother (aged 3⅓ years) lived in the same single-family home prior to their involvement with protective services.

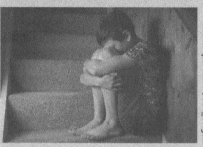

©iStockphoto.com/Ben_Gingell

Henry's home had never been a happy one. Mr. Evans worked several part-time jobs to make ends meet. The family never seemed to have enough money and, consequently, were forced to rent a small, two-bedroom home in a bad neighborhood. Mrs. Bryers had also worked part-time before the birth of her most recent baby. Now a stay-at-home mom, Mrs. Bryers struggles to keep up with household tasks and the responsibilities of raising four children during her husband's frequent absences. The couple's relationship was strained by Mr. Evan's alcohol use and Mrs. Bryers's history of anxiety and chronic stomach ailments that often left her incapacitated. The couple frequently argued and occasionally hit and shoved each other. Their loud altercations were well known to neighbors and (on two occasions) the police.

Several months ago, Henry and his siblings were removed from his parent's custody following a particularly violent interaction. The police report indicated that Henry's father hit his mother while intoxicated. The attack left Mrs. Bryers with a large gash on her forehead. Unfortunately, Henry and his siblings witnessed the injury. They also saw Mrs. Bryers defend herself by shooting a handgun at her husband. Mrs. Bryers had poor aim and left a large bullet hole in the living room wall. Henry and his sisters and brother were subsequently removed from the home.

Henry adjusted poorly to living with his maternal aunt, Jocelyn. After several weeks of separation from his parents and three siblings, Henry was sad and emotionally withdrawn. According to his aunt, Henry acted like "he had lost all sense of joy." He did not want to play games or interact with other children in the neighborhood. Although Henry was known as a troublemaker before the incident, his behavior at school worsened. He seemed to have no attention span, could not concentrate on assignments, and was often moody, irritable, and easily upset by others. On two occasions, Henry reacted aggressively to classmates—once by biting and the second time by hitting a classmate on the playground.

Jocelyn was most troubled by Henry's sleep problems. Henry often had problems falling asleep and would frequently ask Jocelyn if he could sleep on the floor of her bedroom at night. He was especially reluctant to sleep by himself at night because he expected "bad things" to happen. (He was initially in bed at the time the incident with his parents occurred.) Henry also experienced nightmares, approximately 2 or 3 times each week. Henry refused to tell Jocelyn about these dreams, claiming that he "didn't want to talk about them." Jocelyn suspected that these dreams involved his parents because Henry said words like "mom," "no," and "stop" in his sleep but she could not be sure.

Henry's father is currently incarcerated for felonious assault. Henry has biweekly, supervised visitation with his mother. However, Henry refuses to visit his mother at their home and insists that he will remain living with his aunt. His social worker says that family reunification is planned for next month.

Discussion Questions

1. What DSM-5 disorder best describes Henry's behavior?

2. How does Henry meet DSM-5 diagnostic criteria for this condition?

3. The case study does not describe Henry's immediate reaction to observing his parents' fight. Is his reaction important to determine his DSM-5 diagnosis?

4. In what way might Henry's functioning *before* witnessing his parents' fight predict his behavior and emotions *after* the incident?

5. What evidence-based interventions might a psychologist use to help Henry?

This case study accompanies the textbook: Weis, R. (2021). *Introduction to abnormal child and adolescent psychology* (4th ed.). Thousand Oaks, CA: Sage. Answers appear in the online instructor resources. Visit **https://sagepub.com**.

CASE STUDY
HAPPY AND YOU KNOW IT

Ten-year-old Darla Daniels rode home on the bus with 25 other children from Dairyland Public School. The bus rolled to a stop because a van blocked the road. Darla looked up as two masked men suddenly entered the bus, brandishing weapons. The gunmen instructed them to leave the bus and enter the unmarked

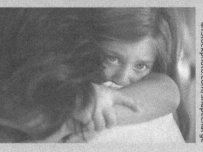

©iStockphoto.com/shapecharge

van with windows painted over. For the next 11 hours, the children cried as the van transported them to an unknown destination.

When the van doors finally opened, the children found themselves in a dark, abandoned quarry. The gunmen ordered the children to climb down a ladder into an opening in the ground. With the aid of a flashlight, they discovered that they were being imprisoned inside a truck that had been buried under several feet of rubble. After all the children entered the truck, the kidnappers retrieved the ladder and placed a metal panel over the opening. After several minutes of shoveling sounds, the children realized they had been buried alive.

The inside of the truck provided no fresh air. The younger children began to cry. The older children wondered if they would ever see their families again. One child bumped the cabin wall, loosening the metal panel and sending dirt and other debris onto their heads. The children panicked, thinking that the ceiling would collapse. Some of the older children tried to distract the younger ones by singing, "If You're Happy and You Know It."

Suddenly, two older boys devised a plan. With much effort, the boys were able to reach a small opening in the ceiling and dig their way out. Many hours later, one of the boys saw the first light of dawn above his head. The children climbed up on each other's shoulders and escaped. The kidnappers were later arrested and imprisoned.

Although no child was seriously hurt, they all experienced social and emotional problems: anxiety attacks, including fear of the dark, difficulty separating from parents, and chronic worry. All of the children also experienced sleep problems or nightmares. Many children engaged in play that resembled the event, such as burying their toy trucks or dolls in the sand. The Dairyland school bus kidnapping provided the first evidence that children could experience psychological problems following a single traumatic event (Terr, 1979, 1983).

Today, most of the survivors of the kidnapping have children of their own (Associated Press, 2020). "The event had a happy ending, but nonetheless, it did damage," reported Darla. "I was extremely terrified for years of strangers and vans. I had endless nightmares, a lifetime of claustrophobia, anxiety and panic attacks. My children never rode the bus and if they had to go on a field trip, I went with them." A second survivor, Jennifer, also described herself as an overprotective mom. "Your children don't get to lead a normal life: to get on the bus, go on a field trip, stay the night with a friend. It's been very difficult." The wife of a third survivor, John, recalled a time when she was singing "If You're Happy and You Know It" to their preschooler. "Honey," John said, "That's not a good song to sing. Can you sing something else?"

Discussion Questions

1. Terr's research with the children who experienced the school bus hijacking showed that young children could experience PTSD. Before that time, PTSD was believed to be an adult disorder, largely experienced by combat veterans. Which DSM-5 PTSD signs or symptoms did these children show?

2. How are the DSM-5 criteria for PTSD in preschool-age children different than the criteria for PTSD in older children, adolescents, and adults?

3. If you were a police officer or other first responder when the children were rescued, how might you use Psychological First Aid to help them?

References

Associated Press. (2020). *James Schoenfeld allowed parole in California school bus hijacking.* Retrieved from March 1, 2020, from https://apnews.com/ea1e affceab6484bbbcb1c71d1cbc21c

Terr, L. (1979). Children of Chowchilla. *Psychoanalytic Study of the Child, 34,* 547–623.

Terr, L. (1983). Chowchilla revisited. *American Journal of Psychiatry, 140,* 1543–1550.

This case study accompanies the textbook: Weis, R. (2021). *Introduction to abnormal child and adolescent psychology* (4th ed.). Thousand Oaks, CA: Sage. Answers appear in the online instructor resources. Visit **https://sagepub.com**.

13

DEPRESSION, SUICIDE, AND SELF-INJURY

Isaac Morgan was an 11-year-old boy brought to the emergency department of our hospital by the police. Earlier that evening, Isaac's mother told Isaac that she would not take him to soccer practice until he cleaned his room. Isaac whined, but Mrs. Morgan insisted. Isaac became belligerent, ran upstairs to his room, and began breaking toys and other objects. His mother 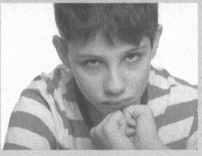 chased him upstairs and ordered him to stop. Isaac began screaming, grabbed a pair of scissors, and waved them at his mother, ordering her to leave him alone. With some difficulty, Mrs. Morgan was able to wrestle the scissors from Isaac's hands. Isaac continued to scream and tried to scratch her with his fingernails. Exasperated and frightened, Mrs. Morgan returned downstairs to call her husband. While she was on the telephone, Isaac began banging his head against his bedroom wall, wailing in a loud voice, "I need to go. I need to go. You can't make me clean my room!" Mrs. Morgan immediately called 911.

Mrs. Morgan provided background information to the psychologist at the hospital. Isaac had a history of violent temper tantrums beginning approximately 5 years ago. At first, the tantrums occurred only at home when Isaac's parents would make him perform a chore or punish him with time out. Later, the tantrums became more violent and arose with little provocation. For example, Isaac would scream and throw objects when he learned that he could not go out to play or when he would lose a game of checkers. Two years ago, Isaac also began showing similar tantrums in class and on the playground at school. Last year, he was suspended for throwing a book at a teacher. This year, he began attending a special education class for students with "emotional disturbance." On average, Isaac tantrums 4 to 5 times per week, with each tantrum lasting between 30 minutes and 2 hours. He seldom showed remorse after he recovered from each tantrum.

When Isaac is not having tantrums, he presents as a disruptive and moody child. His mother describes him as "irritable, grouchy, or cranky" most of the time. His father calls him "a pain in the ass who is set off by the smallest setbacks or disappointments." Both parents admit that Isaac has had long-standing problems with oppositional and defiant behavior. "Isaac never listens to us and seems to take delight in pushing our buttons," said his father.

Isaac showed early delays in gross motor skills (e.g., walking), fine motor skills (e.g., using utensils), and spoken language. In school, he showed deficits in reading acquisition and math. His academic problems were compounded by problems with hyperactivity and impulsivity beginning at age 4 and inattention and poor concentration at age 6. He was formally diagnosed with ADHD at age 7 and has been prescribed a litany of stimulant medications that have yielded only limited benefits.

Last year, a psychiatrist diagnosed Isaac with bipolar I disorder because of his problems with irritability, distractibility, and talkativeness combined with his recurrent (and often violent) tantrums or "rages." Isaac has no family history of bipolar disorder and lithium had little effect on his behavior.

Isaac's parents report that Isaac's behavior has placed considerable strain on their marriage. They frequently argue about him and have contemplated separating. They also admit that they often neglect their other two boys, Noah (7) and Asher (4), because Isaac demands so much attention. Mrs. Morgan reported a history of major depression that has worsened considerably in the past 2 years. Mr. Morgan reported a mixture of anxiety, insomnia, and alcohol use problems.

Isaac was reluctant to talk with the psychologist and provide additional information regarding his thoughts and feelings. The psychologist offered to meet with him individually the next day. Isaac replied, "Why? There's nothing wrong with me."

Discussion Questions

1. What DSM-5 disorder best describes Isaac's current problems with irritability and tantrums?

2. Provide a rationale for your primary diagnosis.

3. Assuming Isaac meets DSM-5 criteria for ADHD, can he also be diagnosed with this disorder?

4. Assuming Isaac meets DSM-5 criteria for oppositional defiant disorder (ODD), can he also be diagnosed with this disorder?

5. Why is bipolar I disorder probably *not* an accurate diagnosis for Isaac?

(Continued)

(Continued)

6. What psychiatric problems is Isaac most at risk for developing in adulthood?

7. What brain areas may be responsible for the problems with emotion regulation shown by children like Isaac?

8. Identify two psychosocial treatments that might be effective for Isaac.

This case study accompanies the textbook: Weis, R. (2021). *Introduction to abnormal child and adolescent psychology* (4th ed.). Thousand Oaks, CA: Sage. Answers appear in the online instructor resources. Visit **https://sagepub.com**.

CASE STUDY
THE NEW KID

Danielle is a 16-year-old high school student who recently moved from a small town in Minnesota to Santa Barbara, California. Danielle's soccer coach referred her to the school psychologist because he was concerned about her sad affect and withdrawn behavior. Although Danielle is a good midfielder and has been on the 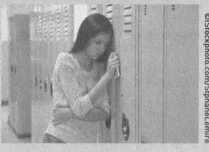 soccer team since transferring to the school last semester, she has repeatedly commented that she "no longer enjoys playing" and feels like she "doesn't fit in" with the other girls on her team. Danielle admitted to problems making friends at her new school. She feels terribly homesick, missing her former classmates and teammates.

Danielle was a straight-A student and star soccer player at her high school in Minnesota. She repeatedly made the high honor roll and started as a center midfielder on both her school varsity soccer team and a competitive travel team during the summer. In California, however, Danielle found her classes much more difficult. Although she studied incessantly, she was unable to earn grades higher than Bs and was struggling to pass language arts. Moreover, she was unable to gain a starting position on her school soccer team, which already had many players who were more talented and experienced than Danielle. Although Danielle put countless hours into practicing, she seldom played more than a few minutes each game and had yet to score or assist in a goal.

The school psychologist asked Danielle to describe a typical school day. Danielle explained that she has a difficult time waking in the morning, can't concentrate on her classes during the day, and usually eats lunch alone. She continued, "After school, I try to get enough energy together to go to soccer practice, but my heart is not in it. Anyway, what's the point? I'm not as good as the other girls on the team and I'll never get to play as much as I did back home."

The school psychologist asked, "Have you thought about getting a tutor, to help you with language arts?"

Danielle replied, "No. It's just no use. I'm no good at anything. I'm a total loser."

"What about friends?" asked the school psychologist. "Have you tried to make friends with the girls on your team?"

Danielle answered, "At first I did. But I could tell that they didn't like me. They already have their own friends. Who wants to be friends with the new kid?"

(Continued)

©iStockphoto.com/StphaneLemire

(Continued)

Discussion Questions

1. What DSM-5 disorder best describes Danielle's behavior?

2. How does Danielle meet diagnostic criteria for this disorder?

3. How might a cognitive therapist, like Aaron Beck, explain Danielle's mood disorder?

4. How might a behavior therapist, like Martin Seligman, explain Danielle's mood disorder?

5. How might an interpersonal therapist, like Myrna Weissman, explain Danielle's mood disorder?

This case study accompanies the textbook: Weis, R. (2021). *Introduction to abnormal child and adolescent psychology* (4th ed.). Thousand Oaks, CA: Sage. Answers appear in the online instructor resources. Visit **https://sagepub.com**.

CASE STUDY
LAST DANCE

Melody O'Neil was born to dance. Her mother enrolled her in ballet at the age of 4. When Melody was 6, she began Irish dance lessons at the insistence of her grandmother who emigrated from Ireland when she was a girl. Melody instantly fell in love with everything about Irish dance: the steps, the music, the incessant practice, 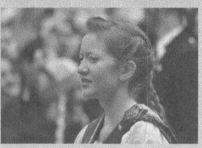 and the close connection it had with her family's ancestry. Melody also proved to be a very good dancer, winning local competitions and being featured in several recitals.

Dance lessons, costumes, and wigs were expensive. So were the entry fees and travel costs associated with competitions. Her mother began working a second, part-time job to help pay for private lessons in addition to group instruction. Her father spent weekends remodeling the family's basement into a dance studio so Melody could practice at home. Melody's younger sisters often were carted to Melody's practices, recitals, and competitions. Melody's room was decorated with Irish paraphernalia, recital brochures, ribbons, and trophies.

Now 15, Melody auditioned for a spot in the best Irish dance company in the region. Although it would place an even greater burden on her family, her parents agreed that if she was going to achieve success as a professional dancer, she needed to be trained by the best instructors. During the audition, Melody gave it her all. Her mother commented afterward, "You danced beautifully—the best I have ever seen you dance. I'm sure you'll get a spot."

Melody's mother was wrong. She was not selected for a spot. The leader of the dance company commented, "Melody is a good dancer, but she doesn't have the skills that we expect from a girl her age."

Melody took the news hard, but not as hard as her parents. Although they did not say so, their actions indicated that they began to regret the sacrifices they made for Melody. Melody's mother quit her second job and cut back on the extra lessons and special recitals for Melody. Both parents seemed to spend more time with the other children in the family. Her dad began coaching one daughter's basketball team; her mother volunteered to lead the other daughter's Girl Scout troop. Melody began to feel less "special" than before and she hated it.

One year later, Melody was referred to counseling after attempting suicide. The police report indicated that she had tried to kill herself by mixing alcohol and her mother's antidepressant medication. Luckily, her younger sister discovered her lying unconscious in her bedroom, and Melody was able to receive medical

(Continued)

(Continued)

treatment. The physician who treated Melody also noticed superficial cuts on her thighs that were likely self-inflicted.

During an interview with a psychologist at the hospital, Melody admitted to severe depression and suicidal ideation with intent to die. "No one loves me anymore," she reported. "My mom and dad sacrificed so much for me—all for nothing. I tried my best, but my best just wasn't good enough. I was a big fish doing well in a small pond, but I couldn't advance beyond that."

For a long while, Melody sobbed into her arm. She added, "My family will be better off without me. They can spend more time with my sisters. Maybe *they* can make something of themselves."

Discussion Questions

1. Use the hopelessness theory of suicide to explain the possible causes of Melody's suicidal behavior.

2. Use the interpersonal-psychological theory of suicide to explain the possible causes of Melody's suicidal behavior.

3. Imagine that you are the psychologist at the hospital who interviews Melody. After Melody stays in the hospital overnight, you decide that she can return home under her parents' supervision. What three components might you include in a safety plan for Melody?

4. Melody's physician prescribes the antidepressant medication Prozac. Her parents are concerned that Prozac could be dangerous for Melody because it might increase her likelihood of suicide. Based on the research data, are her parents' worries justified?

5. How might a therapist use dialectical behavior therapy to help Melody?

This case study accompanies the textbook: Weis, R. (2021). *Introduction to abnormal child and adolescent psychology* (4th ed.). Thousand Oaks, CA: Sage. Answers appear in the online instructor resources. Visit **https://sagepub.com**.

14

PEDIATRIC BIPOLAR DISORDERS AND SCHIZOPHRENIA

CASE STUDY

THE JOKER

Nolan Mitchell was a 9-year-old boy referred to the psychologist at his school for "inappropriate behavior" in his fourth-grade classroom. Earlier that day, Nolan had been sent to the principal's office for repeatedly making "animal noises" in class.

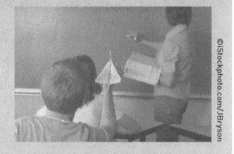

"Nolan's snorting, chirping, and grunting were finally too much," his teacher reported. "I'm not sure what's gotten into him lately. In the last few months, he's gone from being an active, but generally compliant, boy to a class clown and troublemaker."

Indeed, Nolan was now known as "the Joker," a moniker given to him by several classmates because of his frequent antics during school. Nolan had a history of hyperactive and inattentive behavior, beginning in preschool. He was always talkative, had a hard time remaining seated during class, and was easily distracted by even minor stimuli. Recently, however, his impulsivity and attention problems at school worsened. Nolan couldn't resist the urge to blurt out funny comments during

(Continued)

(Continued)

class, make rude noises, disrupt classmates' activities, and perform various stunts or pranks (e.g., attempting to climb out the classroom window onto the building's roof; releasing the class's pet turtles in the bathroom). Most salient were Nolan's frequent laughs, giggles, and chuckles, sometimes for no apparent reason.

None of Nolan's antics were deliberately malicious or disrespectful to others. His teacher commented, "When I reprimand Nolan, he's very apologetic. He's a good boy deep down. It's just that he loses control a lot."

Nolan's mother reported similar problems with his behavior and emotion regulation at home. Approximately 3 weeks ago, Nolan began experiencing increased difficulty attending to his schoolwork, remaining seated at dinner, and carrying on quiet conversations with family members.

"He began talking very rapidly—so fast that we often had to ask him to repeat himself," recalled his mother. "He was like a recording being played at twice the speed. It was also sometimes difficult for us to follow his train of thought. He's always had trouble staying on topic, but now it was worse than usual. It was like he couldn't focus at all."

Most problematic was a change in Nolan's sleep. He would resist going to bed at his usual time, claiming that he was not tired. "I caught him playing on his iPod, assembling Legos, or coloring several hours after he was supposed to be asleep," his mother reported. "When I told him to go to bed, he became very upset and cried for an hour in his room, claiming that he couldn't."

Nolan also woke early in the morning, approximately 2 or 3 hours before the rest of his family. Although he averaged only 4 or 5 hours of sleep each night, he never reported fatigue. Nolan's change in sleep-wake cycle was accompanied by a change in mood. His energetic, high-rate behavior was sometimes peppered by instances of crankiness and irritability.

"We noticed that little things would set him off," recalled his stepfather. "I'd tell him to help with the dishes or to turn off the TV and eat dinner, and he'd become argumentative. On two occasions, he swore right in front of us, which he has never done before."

Nolan's mother added, "He's also had a couple of meltdowns: once after basketball practice when I told him that we didn't have time to stay late, and once in the morning, when I told him that I wouldn't drive him to school and he needed to take the bus. Nolan screamed, kicked at the walls and furniture, and generally behaved like a 2-year-old. He didn't settle down for hours and only because he was exhausted."

Although Nolan was a young boy, he had an extensive psychiatric history. He was diagnosed with ADHD at age 6. His symptoms were managed relatively well with stimulant medication, although he still showed overactivity at school and problems sustaining his attention on homework. Nolan also had an episode of depression during his parents' separation and divorce when he was 7. His depressive episode lasted approximately 9 months and was characterized by sadness, a lack of interest in play and sports, social withdrawal, and extreme irritability and temper tantrums. The episode resolved without treatment.

More recently, Nolan began reporting problems with chronic worrying: about school, friends, sports, his family—all sorts of topics. His increase in worrying was accompanied by more frequent headaches, stomachaches, and other vague physical complaints that sometimes caused him to miss school. Nolan's problems with anxiety predated the onset of his sleep problems by approximately 1 year. A selective serotonin reuptake inhibitor (SSRI), prescribed by his pediatrician, reduced the frequency of his worrying but seemed to exacerbate the severity of his hyperactivity, impulsivity, and inattention. His parents also noticed that the medication immediately preceded the onset of Nolan's antics at school.

During an interview, Nolan's mother reported long-standing problems with generalized anxiety, recurrent panic attacks, and depression. She also admitted to a history of alcohol use problems. She continued to participate in Alcoholics Anonymous meetings to maintain sobriety. Nolan's biological father has a history of bipolar disorder that required hospitalization on two occasions because of self-injury.

During an initial (albeit brief) interview with the school psychologist, Nolan said that he was sorry for disrupting class. He had problems remaining seated, was repeatedly distracted by noises and other activity in the hallway outside the office, and talked very rapidly. Nolan denied feelings of sadness and described his mood as "good." When asked if he had noticed a change in his behavior in the past few weeks, Nolan responded, "I guess so. I never used to get into so much trouble."

Discussion Questions

1. What DSM-5 disorder best describes Nolan's behavior?

2. How does Nolan meet DSM-5 diagnostic criteria for this condition?

3. If Nolan did not have a history of major depression, could he still receive the same primary diagnosis that you assigned in question 1 above?

4. Why doesn't Nolan meet diagnostic criteria for bipolar II disorder?

5. Is there evidence that Nolan exhibits psychotic features during his mood disturbance?

6. Is there evidence that Nolan exhibits mixed features in his mood disturbance?

7. Can Nolan also be diagnosed with ADHD?

8. Why is disruptive mood dysregulation disorder (DMDD) probably *not* the best diagnostic label for Nolan?

9. Based on the results of the Course and Outcome of Bipolar Youth (COBY) study, what is Nolan's prognosis if he participates in treatment?

10. What medications might be effective for Nolan?

11. What psychosocial treatments might you recommend for Nolan and his parents?

This case study accompanies the textbook: Weis, R. (2021). *Introduction to abnormal child and adolescent psychology* (4th ed.). Thousand Oaks, CA: Sage. Answers appear in the online instructor resources. Visit **https://sagepub.com**.

CASE STUDY
GOD'S SERVANT

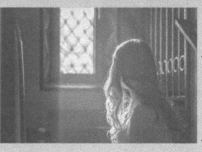

Our patient was an unidentified adolescent girl brought to the emergency department of the hospital by the police. She received lacerations from a physical altercation with a homeless man in a city park. An initial mental status examination indicated that the girl was not oriented to time or place; furthermore, she refused to provide her name or other identifying information. Instead, the girl remained unresponsive, lying in the hospital bed, wrapped in blankets and curled into a ball like a pill-bug. Witnesses saw the girl attempting to care for homeless adults in the park. Although one man resisted her help, the girl insisted on providing it. One thing led to another, a fight ensued, and the girl sustained minor injuries to her arms and right leg.

Identification found in the girl's coat revealed that her name was Julianna McCall, a 16-year-old high school student from a nearby, affluent suburb. Her parents were contacted. They immediately drove to the hospital and provided additional background information.

Julianna had disappeared approximately 24 hours earlier. Her parents were surprised when she did not come home immediately from school on Friday afternoon, because she seldom left the house and never socialized with friends on weekends. After several hours, they filed a police report, organized an informal search, and spent the night worried sick about their daughter.

Julianna was born full-term. Although her gestation and delivery were unremarkable, she showed delays in gross motor, fine motor, and expressive language skills. By the time she began school, she had largely caught up with her peers. Throughout primary school, she was generally well liked, earned average grades, and participated in several extracurricular activities such as swimming, 4-H, and horseback riding.

Julianna showed problems transitioning to high school, however. She became "moody" at home and began spending less time with her parents and younger siblings. She dropped out of many activities, except for horseback riding (which she loved), and withdrew from her former friends. By her sophomore year in high school, Julianna was a recluse. She would usually come home from school, lock herself in her room, and occupy her time watching movies or perusing social media. Her grades in school plummeted. Her parents met with the school guidance counselor who suggested that Julianna's difficulties reflected "typical adolescent adjustment problems."

Not so. Within the last few months, Julianna's functioning changed dramatically. She was reluctant to attend school, rarely left her room, and never interacted with family members. When she did attend school, her teachers described her as "withdrawn and emotionally distant." On at least two occasions, she missed entire school days, hiding in the school bathroom or a supply closet.

Perhaps more concerning was Julianna's increased preoccupation with religion. Although her family was not very religious, Julianna spent much of her time praying. When she did talk to others, she made comments about "saving her soul," "resisting the devil," and "helping God's children." Her speech was noticeably rapid and her train of thought became difficult to follow. Once, her father directly confronted her about her preoccupation with praying. Julianna responded in an angry manner, claiming that he would not lead her astray from her "work" and that she was "God's servant."

Julianna was admitted to the hospital for observation. The next day, she was responsive and answered questions from the psychologist. In a lethargic and unemotional manner, she reported that she went to the park "to help the homeless men and women as expiation for her sins."

"What did you do that was sinful?" asked the psychologist.

"Everything I do is sinful," Julianna replied. "That is what he tells me. That's what he's telling me now."

"You hear a voice now?" asked the psychologist.

Julianna's eyes were downcast as she explained, "It's more like a whisper. Right now it's quiet but it gets louder sometimes."

"What does it say?" asked the psychologist.

"It says," Julianna paused and then continued, "It says that my soul is evil, that others can smell its evilness, and that I am going to go to hell."

"Whose whisper is it?" asked the psychologist.

For the first time during the interview, Juliana looked into the psychologist's eyes, allowed a small tear to trickle down her cheek, and answered, "The devil's."

Discussion Questions

1. What DSM-5 disorder best describes Julianna's behavior?

2. How does Julianna meet diagnostic criteria for this condition?

3. Many youths show premorbid or prodromal signs and symptoms prior to their first psychotic episode. What premorbid or prodromal signs and symptoms did Julianna experience?

4. What is Julianna's prognosis?

5. What two brain pathways are implicated in schizophrenia?

6. What is attenuated psychosis syndrome? Did Julianna meet diagnostic criteria for this condition immediately prior to her first psychotic episode?

7. Is medication effective to help youths like Julianna? What are some limitations of medication as a first-line therapy?

8. How might psychotherapy be used to help Julianna and her family?

This case study accompanies the textbook: Weis, R. (2021). *Introduction to abnormal child and adolescent psychology* (4th ed.). Thousand Oaks, CA: Sage. Answers appear in the online instructor resources. Visit **https://sagepub.com**.

15

FEEDING AND EATING DISORDERS

Demarco Johnson was a beautiful baby who was born approximately 5 weeks premature. His mother had a difficult pregnancy with preeclampsia beginning at 32 weeks gestation. She experienced high blood pressure, severe headaches, nausea, and weight loss. She needed to be hospitalized and delivered Demarco early. Demarco was 5 pounds, 2 ounces at birth (low birth weight) with low blood oxygen levels.

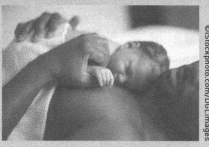

©iStockphoto.com/DGLimages

After Demarco was medically stable, his mother attempted to feed him by breast and bottle. Although he was able to latch onto the nipple, his suck reflex was very weak and he was unable to ingest sufficient nutrition. After 2 days of attempted feeding, his mother, nurses, and lactation expert grew more worried about his ability to eat. Mrs. Johnson grew increasingly frustrated with his passivity. By the time Mrs. Johnson was scheduled to be discharged, the nurse had written NPO in large letters on Demarco's patient board. The abbreviation stood for the Latin words *nil per os* ("nothing by mouth").

Demoralized, Mr. and Mrs. Johnson reluctantly agreed to feed Demarco by an NG (nasogastric) tube, which is a long tube that delivers nutrients through the baby's nostrils, down his esophagus, and into his stomach. When Demarco failed to gain sufficient weight by his 1-month checkup, his parents agreed to switch to a more permanent G (gastric) tube that delivered food directly into Demarco's stomach through a button-like opening in his abdomen. Although Demarco remained at approximately the 15th percentile for weight, he was able to ingest sufficient nutrition through this method (Milano, Chatoor, & Kerzner, 2019).

The main drawback with Demarco's G tube was that he never learned to eat solids. When he was 7 months old, his parents attempted to feed him liquefied and pureed foods orally: rice cereal with formula, apricots, peas, applesauce. Demarco resisted everything. Initially, he accepted food into his mouth, but then thrust the food out with his tongue. When his parents insisted that he eat, Demarco became obstinate. He would arch his back, turn his head, flail his arms, and cry uncontrollably. If he ingested a little food, Demarco would gag or spit up. Eventually, the mere sight of the spoon, bowl, and bib caused him to panic.

Now a 30-month-old toddler, Demarco continues to receive nearly all his nutrients and fluids by G tube. He continues to lag behind other toddlers in weight (26 pounds). His pediatrician recommended surgery and behavior therapy to help wean him off the G tube, but his parents are not sure he (or they) are ready.

Discussion Questions

1. What DSM-5 disorder best describes Demarco's eating behavior?

2. How does Demarco's resistance toward solid foods illustrate Chatoor's (2009) transactional model for feeding disorders?

3. How might classical conditioning be used to partially explain Demarco's refusal to eat solid foods?

4. How might negative reinforcement be used to partially explain Demarco's refusal to eat solid foods?

5. How might exposure therapy be used to treat Demarco?

6. How might a behavior therapist help Demarco and his parents overcome his problem with feeding?

Reference

Chatoor, I. (2009). *Diagnosis and treatment of feeding disorders in infants, toddlers, and young children*. Washington, DC: National Center for Infants, Toddlers, and Families.

Milano, K., Chatoor, I., & Kerzner, B. (2019). A functional approach to feeding difficulties in children. *Current Gastroenterology Reports, 21*, 51–59.

This case study accompanies the textbook: Weis, R. (2021). *Introduction to abnormal child and adolescent psychology* (4th ed.). Thousand Oaks, CA: Sage. Answers appear in the online instructor resources. Visit **https://sagepub.com**.

CASE STUDY
THE APPLE DOESN'T FALL FAR

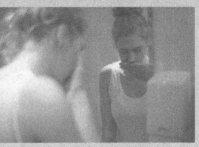

©iStockphoto.com/
KatarzynaBialasiewicz

Miranda Richeson was a 16-year-old girl referred to our eating disorders clinic for assessment and inpatient treatment. Two days ago, Miranda had passed out during physical education class from malnutrition and dehydration. The hospital report indicated that Miranda was significantly underweight compared to girls her height and age, lacked sufficient hydration, and had an electrolyte imbalance. After she was medically stable, they released Miranda to her mother's supervision and set up an intake appointment at our clinic.

Miranda presented as an extremely attractive, well-kempt girl. Perhaps her most striking features were her height (5 feet, 8 inches) and stylish clothes that hung on her frame. Although Miranda reported her mood as "fine," her general disposition seemed to be one of irritability. She resented being questioned by the psychologist. Miranda tended to answer questions using curt, one- or two-word utterances with her eyes fixed on the floor. Occasionally, she glanced at the psychologist and narrowed her eyes with a mixture of scorn and contempt. Her speech suggested above-average intelligence and ample vocabulary, supporting her mother's report that she was an honors student. Thought content focused largely on her desire to leave the treatment facility and return home, feelings of anger toward her mother who insisted that she receive treatment, and preoccupation with friends "back home." When asked specifically about her weight, Miranda reported a preoccupation with her appearance and a desire for perfection. Her insight was poor; although Miranda recognized the need for medical treatment after she passed out during school, she said inpatient treatment was "a big waste of time and money." Nevertheless, Miranda agreed to a "trial run" at the facility for 2 weeks.

Miranda eventually admitted to a history of bingeing and purging beginning approximately 2 years ago, when she was 14. At that time, she had moved from her local public junior high school to a new, private college preparatory school near her mother's workplace in the city. Although Miranda was an excellent student and had many friends at her old school, she initially had difficulty performing well academically and fitting in socially.

Miranda began dieting in order to lose weight. Although she was never overweight, she often felt guilty when she would indulge in pizza, ice cream, and chocolate. Miranda lacked the willpower to sustain her diets for long. After breaking a diet, she would give in to despair, indulge, and regret her weakness later. Several of her new friends introduced her to purging as a means to avoid weight gain. Miranda soon learned that purging not only allowed her to avoid gaining weight, it also allowed her to reduce feelings of guilt for occasionally indulging in her favorite foods. Eventually, she developed a pattern of bingeing and purging that occurred several times per week. She felt out of control, emotionally vulnerable, and guilty for hiding her bingeing and purging from her family.

Miranda's parents knew Miranda had an eating problem, but they never raised their concerns with her. Mrs. Richeson had a history of bulimia in college. "I could see myself in Miranda," she said. "All of the insecurity, the need for perfection, the lack of control. I felt that way for years. Some of her eating habits are probably my fault. Before I got help, I used to always diet and was obsessed with calories. It probably rubbed off on Miranda."

Discussion Questions

1. What DSM-5 disorder best describes Miranda's behavior?

2. How does Miranda meet diagnostic criteria for that disorder?

3. How might a clinician differentiate between the various eating disorders?

4. Identify several health-related problems that Miranda may experience because of her maladaptive eating behavior.

5. How might a psychologist use the cognitive–behavioral model for eating disorders to explain the cause and maintenance of Miranda's problematic eating?

6. How might a psychologist use the tripartite influence model to explain the cause and maintenance of Miranda's problematic eating?

7. How might a psychologist use interpersonal theory to explain the cause and maintenance of Miranda's problematic eating?

8. Identify one way a psychologist might help Miranda, according to (1) cognitive–behavioral theory, (2) the tripartite influence model, and (3) interpersonal theory, respectively.

This case study accompanies the textbook: Weis, R. (2021). *Introduction to abnormal child and adolescent psychology* (4th ed.). Thousand Oaks, CA: Sage. Answers appear in the online instructor resources. Visit **https://sagepub.com**.

HEALTH-RELATED DISORDERS AND PEDIATRIC PSYCHOLOGY

"My son has a problem controlling his bladder."

That is how Mrs. Handler began our first session. "I thought I might explain the situation to you first, before you interview Lawrence himself," she continued. "He'd probably be very embarrassed if he was in the room with us."

"Lawrence is 10 years old. He's a great kid. He's excellent in just about any sport he plays. He's extraverted, has an infectious smile, and loves to play with his little brothers. The only problem is his accidents."

"Tell me about them," I said.

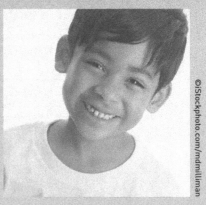

©iStockphoto.com/mdmilliman

Mrs. Handler continued, "My husband and I call him 'Little Late Larry.' He'll be playing a game, or watching TV, or doing something else in the house. Then, he'll get this sudden urge to go. He'll rush over to the bathroom and not make it in time. The funny thing is, when he does wet himself, he doesn't tend to go very much."

"Do you mean he doesn't void much urine when he has an accident?" I asked.

"Yes. Well sometimes he does. But usually it's just enough that it is noticeable."

"Does he wet at night too?" I asked.

"Yes. He wets about 2 or 3 nights a week. We've tried to use a urine alarm to get him to stop, but it hasn't helped. Lawrence wakes up when he wets the bed even without the alarm."

"And at night, when he has an accident, does he also void only a little amount of urine or does he soak the bed?" I asked.

Mrs. Handler responded, "It's usually just enough to wake him up. He's such a good kid. He runs to the bathroom and empties whatever is left, and he even helps us clean up. Bill (his father) and I let him wear disposable underpants to help manage."

I commented, "If it's okay with you, I'd like to talk with Lawrence to get his perspective on this problem. I'd also like to talk with his pediatrician, to make sure there's no medication or illness that might be causing it. How does that sound?"

Discussion Questions

1. How does Lawrence meet DSM-5 diagnostic criteria for enuresis?

2. When does bedwetting become a disorder that merits treatment?

3. What kind of enuresis does Lawrence likely have? Why is knowing his kind of enuresis important?

4. Approximately how many children Lawrence's age experience enuresis?

5. What are the two primary causes for Lawrence's type of nocturnal enuresis?

6. Lawrence also wets during the day. Why do most boys show daytime wetting?

7. Imagine that you were Lawrence's therapist. Outline a psychosocial treatment plan to decrease his daytime wetting.

8. What medication might be used to treat Lawrence? What are the limitations of medication to treat enuresis?

This case study accompanies the textbook: Weis, R. (2021). *Introduction to abnormal child and adolescent psychology* (4th ed.). Thousand Oaks, CA: Sage. Answers appear in the online instructor resources. Visit **https://sagepub.com**.

CASE STUDY

AN EMBARRASSING PROBLEM

Brad was referred to our out-patient clinic by his school guidance counselor. Brad, a cute fourth-grader, was having problems with teasing.

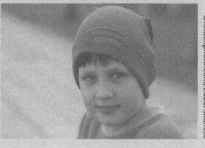

"To put it bluntly, Brad has fecal incontinence," the guidance counselor explained. "He often smells very badly, but I don't think he's even aware of it. The more polite kids in his class simply avoid him. The less polite kids make fun of him behind his back."

One week later, Brad's mother met with me in my office. She explained the situation.

"It's ironic. Brad has always had problems with constipation. As a preschooler, I'd need to use laxative suppositories to help him go. His stool would be very hard and it would be so painful. He'd sit on the toilet and cry. He began avoiding the toilet, probably because he hurt so much."

"So, what's the problem now?" I asked.

Brad's mother responded, "Now, it's the opposite problem. Brad has accidents throughout the day, almost every day. It's usually just a little bit, but it's watery and . . . it doesn't smell so good."

I questioned, "So what have you tried to do to solve the problem?"

She replied, "At first, I tried over-the-counter medication for diarrhea. That didn't work at all. I actually think it made the problem worse. Then, I tried rewarding him for each day he didn't have an accident, but there were so few of them. Then, I started punishing him—taking away privileges—whenever he had an accident. But, honestly, this just made him upset and didn't correct the problem. I think he's just gotten in the habit of having these accidents. He doesn't seem to even realize when he has to go. He doesn't seem to care."

"Brad has a really common, but really embarrassing, problem," I said. "His colon is stretched out and flabby, like a boxer who's taken a beating for many years and is now old and out of shape. We need to get it back into shape so that it can do its job."

Brad's mother replied, "Okay. Whatever it takes."

Discussion Questions

1. How does Brad meet DSM-5 criteria for encopresis?

2. When does soiling become a disorder that merits treatment?

3. Does Brad show primary or secondary encopresis? Why is this distinction important?

4. Approximately how many children Brad's age experience encopresis? How many children with encopresis also have enuresis?

5. What is probably the cause of encopresis? (How might learning theory be used to explain Brad's symptoms?)

6. Imagine that you were Brad's therapist. Outline a psychosocial treatment plan to decrease his encopresis.

7. Why is it important to refer Brad to a pediatrician prior to psychosocial treatment?

This case study accompanies the textbook: Weis, R. (2021). *Introduction to abnormal child and adolescent psychology* (4th ed.). Thousand Oaks, CA: Sage. Answers appear in the online instructor resources. Visit **https://sagepub.com**.

CASE STUDY
SURPRISES

David was a 7-year-old boy who was referred to our outpatient clinic for children with elimination disorders. One day each week, a team of psychologists and pediatricians met with children experiencing enuresis or encopresis and their families. We assessed children's problems with elimination, arrived at a diagnosis, and provided recommendations for treatment so the family could get started correcting the problem right away. David was different from most of the kids we tended to see.

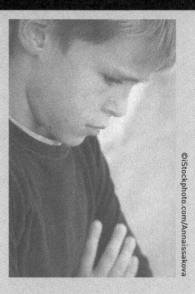

©iStockphoto.com/Annaissakova

"The problem began about 6 months ago," his mother explained. "I was doing the laundry in the basement of our house. I noticed a funny smell and then I saw it. Somebody had defecated in the middle of the pile of dirty clothes. I must have screamed or something. All of the kids came running—all except David. It didn't take long to figure out who the culprit was."

I asked, "Did this happen again?"

She continued, "I punished him pretty hard. He's always been a bit of a troublemaker, but nothing like this! Everything was fine for a while, and then it occurred twice in 1 week. Well, to be honest, I only *noticed* his droppings twice in 1 week—I am not really sure when he left them. I found both of them in the basement, one in the basement shower (which we rarely use) and one in the closet that holds the hot water heater."

"How did you respond?" I asked.

"I was livid," she replied. "How could he do such a thing? I spanked him and took away all of his games and privileges. I was really worried he would start doing this at school!"

"Does he ever have accidents, like soil his pants or wet the bed?" I questioned.

She answered, "No. He's never had problems with soiling or wetting like that. He's a pretty healthy kid. I just don't know what to do. I've got three kids at home and David's the oldest, but he's the one acting like a baby! It's hard enough being a single mom and now I have to deal with this."

"It sounds like you have a lot on your plate. Do you have anyone who can help you?" I asked.

She replied, "Not since their dad left several months ago. I suppose I could ask my sister to help, but she's got kids of her own."

Discussion Questions

1. How does David meet DSM-5 diagnostic criteria for encopresis?

2. When does soiling become a disorder that merits treatment?

3. Does David show primary or secondary encopresis? Why is this distinction important?

4. Approximately how many children David's age experience encopresis? How many children with encopresis also have enuresis?

5. What is the cause of David's encopresis?

6. What other symptoms or comorbid disorders might you want to investigate in David?

7. Imagine that you were David's therapist. Outline a psychosocial treatment plan to decrease his encopresis.

This case study accompanies the textbook: Weis, R. (2021). *Introduction to abnormal child and adolescent psychology* (4th ed.). Thousand Oaks, CA: Sage. Answers appear in the online instructor resources. Visit **https://sagepub.com**.

CASE STUDY

ENFAMIL AND INSOMNIA

"If I hear another mom talk about how her baby is sleeping through the night, I am going to scream!"

Mrs. Drumm brought her 1-year-old son, Benedict, to his pediatrician because of chronic insomnia. His pediatrician had examined Benedict and determined that there was nothing medically wrong with him. Consequently, she suggested that

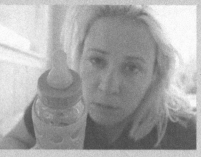

©iStockphoto.com/Lisa5201

Mrs. Drumm consult a pediatric psychologist to help with her son's sleep problems.

Mrs. Drumm continued, "Every night it's the same song and dance. He doesn't want to go to sleep unless we carry him in our arms and feed him. When he was a newborn, it was not a big deal. I would support him with my right arm and hold the bottle for him with my left. Then, when he got older, he would insist on holding the bottle. But, when he starts to drift off, he drops the bottle and wakes up. Then, we have to start the whole routine again. Also, he's getting to be *so heavy*. Do you see these?"

Mrs. Drumm rolled up the sleeve of her right arm, displaying her bicep. She said, "Pretty nice arms for a 38-year-old woman don't you think? The problem is my right arm is bigger around than my left. And I can't sit down. I need to hold him and feed him while walking around the room. If I stop walking or sit down, he wakes up again crying."

"It sounds exhausting!" I said.

She continued, not seeming to hear my comment. "Then, when Ben wakes in the middle of the night, I have to do the same thing all over. He won't go to sleep on his own."

"What would you like to be different?" I asked.

Mrs. Drumm rolled her eyes and replied, "You've got to be kidding me? What do I want to be different? I want to get some sleep! I want this kid to sleep through the night like a normal kid his age. I'm too old for this."

Discussion Questions

1. How does Ben meet DSM-5 diagnostic criteria for insomnia disorder?

2. When does a child's sleep problem become a disorder that merits treatment?

3. At what age do most infants go to sleep on their own and sleep through the night? Is Ben's behavior typical for a 12-month-old?

4. How many hours of sleep should Ben get, if he is typically developing?

5. How might learning theory be used to explain Ben's insomnia?

6. Imagine that you are the therapist for Ben and his mother. How might improved sleep hygiene help reduce Ben's insomnia?

7. How might planned ignoring improve Ben's sleep?

8. Some parents are unable to used planned ignoring with their infants or toddlers. What alternative treatment might you recommend to Ben and his mother?

9. How effective are behavioral interventions to treat infant insomnia?

This case study accompanies the textbook: Weis, R. (2021). *Introduction to abnormal child and adolescent psychology* (4th ed.). Thousand Oaks, CA: Sage. Answers appear in the online instructor resources. Visit **https://sagepub.com**.

©iStockphoto.com/Ben_Gingell

CASE STUDY

THOUGHTS BEFORE BEDTIME

Alex Molnar was a 15-year-old boy who was referred to the sleep disorders clinic of our hospital because of insomnia. For the past 6 months, Alex has experienced problems falling asleep at night. His insomnia had an insidious onset and has grown progressively worse, especially in the past 2 months. Initially, Alex would toss and 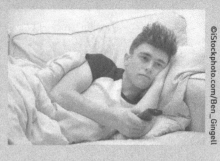 turn in bed, finally falling asleep after an hour-long struggle to rest. Currently, Alex spends many hours, several nights each week, trying to fall asleep. Needless to say, his sleep problems have caused him considerable frustration.

"We tried to get an appointment for the sleep clinic over 6 weeks ago," explained Alex's mother. "I noticed Alex acting like a zombie most of the time. I had to yell at him to get him out of bed in the morning. He'd often be late for the bus and I'd have to drive him to school. Then, when he'd get home, he'd only want to lounge on the couch or watch TV. He was crabby all of the time."

Alex's father added, "What really prompted us to seek help was his performance in school. We noticed a drop in his grades from last year, even in subjects that he used to enjoy. At first, we attributed this drop in grades to problems transitioning from middle school to high school. But when we talked with Alex's math teacher, she commented about his concentration problems and drowsiness at school. She thought Alex might be depressed or have ADHD."

Alex readily admitted to having insomnia. He said that he typically went to bed between 10:00 and 11:30 p.m. Initially, he would feel exhausted when his head hit the pillow. However, soon after laying down, his mind would fill with events that occurred that day. Alex admitted to disproportionately reflecting on bad events: things he said to friends that he later regretted, mistakes he made on tests, or silly things he did that caused embarrassment. He would often chastise himself, thinking, "How could I have been so stupid?" These thoughts caused muscle tension and "a warm feeling in his chest" that made him toss and turn in his bed.

Eventually, his thoughts would turn to the next day: homework that he still needed to complete before class, an important cross-country meet, his dad's chronic health problems. As he thought about each problem, both little hassles and major stressors, Alex felt more helpless. "It's like I'm running in a narrow valley and the cliffs on each side are closing in on me. I can feel tightness in my body, in my chest, everywhere. At that point, I tell myself, 'You've got to get to sleep. It's midnight already and you need to get up at 6:30 for school.'"

Of course, statements like these never helped. Frustrated and angry with himself, Alex would often leave his bedroom, have a snack, and watch a video. YouTube distracted him from his worries, eventually lulling him to sleep. Coffee in the morning, two or three sodas during the day, and Red Bull after school would help him through the next day.

A medical examination revealed no health problems that might cause Alex's sleep disorder. Furthermore, Alex was not taking any medication. The neurologist suggested that his family try a psychosocial intervention before participating in a formal sleep study.

Discussion Questions

1. How does Alex meet DSM-5 diagnostic criteria for insomnia disorder?

2. Does Alex meet criteria for any other mental disorder that might exacerbate his insomnia?

3. Identify three cognitive distortions that might contribute to Alex's excessive worrying and insomnia.

4. What cognitive interventions might be useful to treat Alex's problems?

5. What behavioral interventions might be useful to treat Alex's problems?

6. What medications might be useful to treat Alex's problems?

This case study accompanies the textbook: Weis, R. (2021). *Introduction to abnormal child and adolescent psychology* (4th ed.). Thousand Oaks, CA: Sage. Answers appear in the online instructor resources. Visit **https://sagepub.com**.

CASE STUDY

DAYTIME FATIGUE

Sixteen-year-old Lindsay was referred to our sleep clinic because of chronic fatigue. Lindsay was a perfectionist. She earned high grades, was a star on the cross-country and track teams, and was popular with classmates. Lindsay was excellent at everything she did—everything except for sleeping.

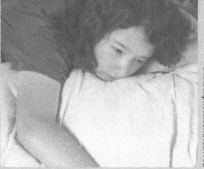

Despite her best efforts, Lindsay had terrible problems going to sleep. Lindsay tried to go to sleep early each night, so that she could get up early the next morning and attend a writing club before school. Often, however, she would lie in bed for hours before finally falling asleep.

"You know what they say. 'Early to bed, early to rise . . . ,'" Lindsay said to me during her first visit. "The problem is, I'll finish studying or come home from some activity and try to get to bed at a reasonable hour. But then, I'd toss and turn in bed, unable to get to sleep."

"What do you do when you can't sleep?" I asked.

"Sometimes I'll get up and watch Netflix for a while or text someone. Usually, I just tell myself, 'C'mon Lind, you know you need to get to sleep,' which makes me even more frustrated because I can't."

I asked, "So what is it like, when you're lying in bed, trying to sleep?"

She answered, "It's like I can't shut off my brain. Instead of relaxing, I'll be thinking of things that happened that day or things that are scheduled for tomorrow."

"I've caught Lindsay up at 2 and 3 in the morning," added her mother.

Lindsay admitted, "Sometimes I watch videos, or have something to eat, or whatever."

Her mother interjected, "The problem is the next day. It's nearly impossible to get her out of bed."

"I want to get up and go to school but just can't," Lindsay reported. "Then, when I get to school, I'm tired all of the time. I have a hard time concentrating."

"How long have you had this problem?" I asked.

"It started when I was in middle school," Lindsay reported. "At first it wasn't too bad, but now it takes me several hours to fall asleep."

"And what about on weekends?" I asked. "Do you have trouble falling asleep on Friday and Saturday nights too?"

"On weekends I know that I don't need to get up early the next day, so I just go to sleep whenever I want, usually about 1 or 2 a.m.," she replied. "Then I sleep most of the next morning."

From the look on her face, I could tell that Lindsay was exasperated. Trying to give her hope, I said, "Maybe I can teach you strategies that could help you get to sleep."

Discussion Questions

1. What DSM-5 sleep-wake disorder best describes Lindsay's condition?

2. How does Lindsay meet diagnostic criteria for this condition?

3. When does an adolescent's sleep problem become a disorder that merits treatment?

4. How many hours of sleep should Lindsay get?

5. Many adolescents show a phase delay in melatonin production after puberty. Why might this be important for Lindsay?

6. What associated symptoms or comorbid disorders would you want to assess prior to treating Lindsay?

7. Imagine that you are Lindsay's therapist. How might you improve Lindsay's sleep hygiene to reduce her sleep problems?

8. How might you use stimulus control and sleep restriction to help Lindsay?

9. How might you use cognitive restructuring to help Lindsay?

10. Most physicians treat pediatric sleep problems with medication. Identify one medication that might be used to help Lindsay fall asleep. What are the side effects of this medication? Would you want your child to take this medication?

This case study accompanies the textbook: Weis, R. (2021). *Introduction to abnormal child and adolescent psychology* (4th ed.). Thousand Oaks, CA: Sage. Answers appear in the online instructor resources. Visit **https://sagepub.com**.

CASE STUDY
A NORMAL LIFE

Caleb Williams was a 10-year-old boy who was referred to a pediatric psychologist at a large children's hospital. Caleb was diagnosed with sickle cell disease shortly after birth and has an extensive medical history related to this condition.

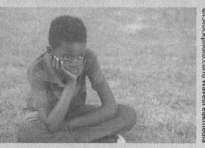

©iStockphoto.com/Wavebreakmedia

Caleb's disorder, hemoglobin SS disease, is a recessive genetic disorder. Both his mother and father were carriers of the disease and Caleb was unlucky enough to inherit the recessive gene from each parent. The disease is especially prevalent among African American children, like Caleb. The disorder causes red blood cells to have a sickle shape, rather than the round shape shown by healthy children. The sickle shape limits the amount of oxygen the blood cells can carry and can cause occlusion (blockages) in children's bloodstream. Sickle cells also have a much shorter lifespan (10–20 days) than healthy red blood cells (120 days), causing children with the disease to experience anemia—that is, a low red blood cell count.

Caleb had experienced the most common effects of sickle cell disease. First, because of his anemia, he was frequently tired and often experienced weakness and fatigue. These symptoms reduced the amount of time that he could play with other children and limited his participation in certain high-intensity sports like basketball and football—two sports that he enjoyed.

Second, Caleb experienced frequent, intense episodes of pain associated with occlusions. Usually, these painful crises occurred in his chest, arms, and legs and lasted for several hours or days. Sometimes, the pain was severe and caused him to miss school and other daily activities. Painful crises often occurred when he was dehydrated (e.g., after running or playing), when he experienced a sudden change in temperature (e.g., playing in the snow, swimming in a cold pool), or when he was under stress (e.g., listening to his parents argue).

Third, Caleb has a history of infections and hospitalizations associated with his disorder. As a toddler, he was diagnosed with acute chest syndrome, a condition characterized by occlusions of vesicles in the lungs, resulting in severe chest pain, coughing, and breathing problems. In preschool, he experienced splenic sequestration syndrome, a serious condition in which his sickle-shaped cells became trapped (i.e., sequestered) in his spleen, causing severe anemia and abdominal pain. He has also been hospitalized on several other occasions because of fevers. Currently, Caleb takes a medication called hydroxyurea (Droxia) that increases hemoglobin and reduces the frequency and intensity of his pain.

During the initial interview with the pediatric psychologist, Caleb's parents reported that Caleb appears irritable and moody. Over the past 6 months, Caleb has shown an increase in lethargy and feelings of hopelessness associated with his sickle cell symptoms. On one occasion, during a painful episode, he commented that "he wished he had never been born." He has also grown angry at being limited in his ability to play sports, run and swim, and do many other physical activities because of chronic fatigue and recurrent pain. Although many of his friends and classmates are sympathetic to his medical problems, his parents have noticed that Caleb is less often invited to others' homes to play.

Caleb's medical condition has also taken its toll on the Williams family more generally. His parents reported very high levels of stress associated with caring for a child with a chronic medical problem. Stressors include (1) making sure that Caleb takes his medication regularly, (2) coordinating Caleb's medical care with his schooling, (3) working with teachers to help Caleb make up missed schoolwork, (4) transporting Caleb to and from medical appointments, (5) paying medical bills, and (6) missing work. Mr. and Mrs. Williams are also concerned that they may be neglecting Caleb's two younger brothers. These stressors have led to increased marital conflict that, in turn, exacerbates Caleb's symptoms.

When interviewed alone, Caleb denied suicidal ideation but readily admitted to feelings of hopelessness and helplessness regarding his illness. "No one understands what it's like . . . " he repeatedly said. "I can't do all the things that I want to do, all the things even my little brothers can do. I can't be a normal kid."

Discussion Questions

1. What is a pediatric psychologist and what are their three main professional activities?

2. What mental health problem(s) might Caleb experience?

3. If you were Caleb's therapist, how might you address adherence in therapy?

4. In what way might behavioral factors (besides adherence) exacerbate Caleb's sickle cell symptoms? How might a therapist address these factors?

5. In what way might emotional factors exacerbate Caleb's sickle cell symptoms? How might a therapist address these factors?

This case study accompanies the textbook: Weis, R. (2021). *Introduction to abnormal child and adolescent psychology* (4th ed.). Thousand Oaks, CA: Sage. Answers appear in the online instructor resources. Visit **https://sagepub.com**.